PRAISE FOR

INFERTILITY JOURNEYS
Finding Your Happy Ending

"Lesley has done a wonderful job in letting her own story guide the reader into new areas where she educates them with stories from other women's experiences. She has a delightful ability to explore, on both a scientific and emotional level, the many options couples have to extend their family. She explores fertility treatments, third-party options, such as egg donors or surrogates, and adoption or childfree living.

The courage it takes to reach deep into your own pain is admirable and Lesley shows a willingness to use this to help others struggling with similar problems.

Infertility Journeys: Finding Your Happy Ending is a must-read for men and women struggling with their own fertility. This book offers inspiration and hope that whatever decisions you make can be right for you."

—L. Michael Kettel, M.D.
San Diego Fertility Center

"Written with self-awareness, honesty, humor, and compassion, *Infertility Journeys: Finding Your Happy Ending* weaves the stories of women and men together with a wealth of information about the medical and psychological processes that patients experience. The book provides not only vivid descriptions of the experience, but important coping tools as well. It truly provides hope for all people experiencing infertility."

—Martha Diamond, Ph.D.
Co-Director, Center for Reproductive Psychology
Co-author, *Unsung Lullabies: Understanding and Coping with Infertility*

"Inspirational, informative, and heart-felt. Using real couples' experiences, this book highlights the ups and downs along the infertility path. A definite must-have for all couples seeking positive guidance and truthful answers to their questions."

—Diana Hoppe, M.D., Board Certified Obstetrician/Gynecologist
Author, *Healthy Sex Drive, Healthy You: What Your Libido Reveals About Your Life*

"*Infertility Journeys: Finding Your Happy Ending* is a heartfelt book which provides a valuable resource for women and men considering infertility treatment. It informs women and men about common terms and infertility procedures used by physicians and alternative practitioners. I recommend this book to my patients, as I think it will bring comfort as well as a better understanding of their choices when faced with infertility. Lesley's writing style is very engaging, and although it is an informative book, it reads like a novel. She has handled a delicate subject with sensitivity, while at the same time imparting a wealth of information in this useful resource."
—Margot J. Aiken, M.D., FRCP, FACE

"Lesley provides much needed information for couples on their fertility journey. *Infertility Journeys: Finding Your Happy Ending* gives excellent advice that will help any couple begin the process of seeking treatment and motivate other couples to continue their journey of starting or growing a family."
—Marc Sklar, LAc, DA (RI), FABORM
Reproductive Wellness

"I highly recommend *Infertility Journeys: Finding Your Happy Ending*, if you've ever felt alone or lost as you struggle with fertility issues. It offers heartfelt stories from many different couples, well-researched information, sound advice, and encouragement for your fertility journey. *Infertility Journeys* also offers a very holistic way to look at your fertility issues, touching upon the mind, body, emotions, and spirituality. The book guides you to discover a balance and to find your own resolution and happy ending."
—Genevieve Siegel, HHP, LMT
Certified Practitioner of Maya Abdominal Therapy

"Lesley Vance writes from the heart and from experience. In her book she chronicles couples like her, who are all dealing, healing and moving forward in their own ways in search of their 'happy endings' – whatever form that might come in. She teaches us that no one should suffer in silence. And much like there are steps in grieving any death…there are steps in dealing with the death of your dream: the child that could have been. She talks about setting limits, letting the tears flow and finding support. The first guidelines I've ever seen for handling miscarriage."
—Kathleen Bade, Journalist & News Anchor
FOX 5 News, KSWB-TV

INFERTILITY JOURNEYS
Finding Your Happy Ending

LESLEY VANCE

DUCK
HILL
PRESS

Encinitas, California

Infertility Journeys: Finding Your Happy Ending may be purchased in bulk for educational, business, fundraising, or sales promotional use. For information, contact Duck Hill Press, P.O. Box 236142, Encinitas, California 92023. Email the publisher at info@DuckHillPress.com.

ISBN 978-0-9829848-0-2
Library of Congress Control Number: 2011931581

Cover design by Chris Vance, www.chrisvancedesign.com
Edited by Marlene Hamerling
Typography by Ryoichi Tsunekawa and Kimberly Geswein

The author and publisher are not engaged in rendering medical or psychological services, and this book is not intended as a guide to diagnose or treat medical or psychological problems. If the reader requires medical, psychological, or other expert assistance, please seek the services of your own physician or certified counselor.

Contact the author at: info@LesleyVance.com
Contact the publisher at: info@DuckHillPress.com

Order online at
www.LesleyVance.com

This book is dedicated to

Brian

the love of my life.

And to all the women and men who bravely shared their infertility journey with me.

Thank you for trusting me with your story.

(All names have been changed to respect each person's privacy.)

TABLE OF CONTENTS

ACKNOWLEDGEMENTS

This book has been a labor of love and there are many people who have supported and encouraged me throughout the writing process. It is with the utmost gratitude that I thank:

Janet Jaffe, Ph.D., for helping me "process" my own loss and unmet expectations; Mom for reading first- and final-drafts to make sure the book was likable; Lisa Prisock for encouraging me to write this book; L. Michael Kettel, M.D., for providing feedback on the book's content and inspiring the title; Martha Diamond, Ph.D.; Marc B. Sklar, LAC, DA; Margot Aiken, M.D.; Diana Hoppe, M.D.; Kathleen Bade; Photographer Gary Lyons; Dr. Lorretta Shughrue; and Genevieve Siegel, HHP.

For their advice, support, and encouragement, I sincerely thank:

My husband, Brian, who walked by my side throughout the ups and downs of putting our experiences on paper. He believed in my vision–to turn our pain into something tangible to offer hope and encouragement to other women and men struggling with pregnancy loss and infertility. He has given me unconditional love and encouragement. Without him this book would have never come to fruition.

My brother, Chris Vance, who is an extraordinary individual–loving, generous and brilliant. He supported me through some of my darkest hours. His support has been invaluable. Chris designed the beautiful cover for my book. He is a gifted artist and I am blessed by his talents (www.ChrisVancePaintings.com).

My friend and mentor, Claudia Jean, who wears many hats acting as my book consultant, content editor, and cheerleader. Throughout my writing journey, she has said, "You're on the right track. Just keep going. This book is meant to be written." There were days when her words were the only thing that kept me writing. (www.ClaudiaJean.com).

My friend, Lynne H. Calkins, CRNP, who is an Ob-Gyn Nurse Practitioner, provided medical editing of my manuscript. She ensured that my manuscript clearly and effectively presented accurate information to my intended audience. Lynne encouraged me throughout my writing process, listening and offering wisdom to help me along my journey.

My copyeditor, Marlene Hamerling, kept me on the straight and narrow with her professional expertise. She fixed my grammatical errors and advised me of sections that needed rewriting for clarity (www. HamerlingAssociates.com).

FOREWORD

The trauma of infertility experienced by people who endure reproductive difficulties can be profound. The layers of loss and grief can be overwhelming, emotionally, mentally and physically, and touch all corners of a person's life. It can cause a severe blow to one's sense of self and place enormous strain on a couple's relationship. People have to assimilate information and make life-altering decisions about treatment while grief-stricken and traumatized. It is a lonely process.

Infertility Journeys: Finding Your Happy Ending by Lesley Vance does much to ease that loneliness. While written as a first-person account of her own reproductive journey, it is far more than another emotional diary of one person's experience. What makes this book stand out is that interwoven through Lesley's personal story, is a wealth of information about the medical and psychological processes that patients experience. She provides vivid descriptions and explanations of the diagnostic work-up by the reproductive endocrinologist, the medical interventions available and the alternative paths to parenthood, such as adoption or surrogacy. She includes important questions that couples should ask both in choosing medical professionals and in making treatment decisions. Perhaps most important, she explores the complex and varied emotional journey of choosing to stop treatment and remain childfree. By including an in-depth discussion of this option, which is rarely talked about, Lesley truly provides hope for all people experiencing infertility—that they have a future, and a very rich and fulfilling future, regardless of whether they become parents.

Infertility Journeys is also unique in that it contains the personal experiences of men, as well as women, interspersing quotes and observations by the author's husband, Brian, as he traveled the road with her. Enhanced by additional stories of other men and women, *Infertility Journeys* provides not only vivid descriptions of the experience, but important coping tools as well. Notably, the author includes holistic activities such as meditation, massage, and acupuncture as methods that can bring enormous relief, and she offers clear and understandable lessons about how to make use of these.

The experience of infertility is life-changing, but it is an experience from which people can heal and grow. Written with self-awareness, honesty, humor, and compassion, *Infertility Journeys: Finding Your Happy Ending* is a welcome addition to the literature.

—Martha Diamond, Ph.D.
Co-Director, Center for Reproductive Psychology
Co-author, *Unsung Lullabies: Understanding and Coping with Infertility*
(St. Martin's Press, 2005) and *Reproductive Trauma: Psychotherapy with Infertility and Pregnancy Loss Clients* (APA Press, 2011)

INTRODUCTION

Lesley Vance has opened her soul and let others into her personal journey through the ups and down of infertility and pregnancy loss. *Infertility Journeys: Finding Your Happy Ending* is a touching, yet educational, book that chronicles Brian and Lesley's own experiences and diverges just enough to provide her own insight into the pitfalls that can be encountered when starting a family. They share the excitement that goes with a couples' decision that it is finally the "right time" to get pregnant. They also share their own heartbreak and disappointment that goes with reproductive loss.

Lesley has done a wonderful job in letting her own story guide the reader into new areas where she educates them with stories from other women's experiences. She has a delightful ability to explore, on both a scientific and emotional level, the many options couples have to extend their family. She explores fertility treatments, third-party options, such as egg donors or surrogates, and adoption or childfree living.

The courage it takes to reach deep into your own pain is admirable and Lesley shows a willingness to use this to help others struggling with similar problems.

If you, or a loved one, are struggling with their own fertility and need the insight that comes with knowing that you are not alone, *Infertility Journeys: Finding Your Happy Ending* will give you inspiration and hope that whatever decisions you make can be right for you.

—L. Michael Kettel, M.D.
San Diego Fertility Center

A flickering dream is the light
at the end of every tunnel.

—Lesley Vance

CHAPTER ONE

normal expectations

My Conception

I've heard the story a thousand times. My mother giggles every time she tells it. It's 1968. I don't know what possessed her, but Mom enrolled in belly dancing classes. For weeks, without my dad knowing, she secretly took lessons on hip bumps, the shimmy and belly rolls. She planned to surprise him with her new skills. One day as dad walked in the door from work, he was stunned to find my mother standing barefoot on the living-room coffee table. He stared in awe at her pink chiffon veil, gold beaded skirt, swaying hip sash ringing with dangling coins and finger cymbals snapping a rhythmic beat. Arabic dance music was bathing the room in mystery as she began to shimmy. I don't know how long she danced. I haven't asked. All I know is that mom swears I was conceived that magical night.

Family

Most of us grow up hearing stories of how babies are made. We discover from our mothers and fathers, grandmothers and grandfathers, aunts and uncles -- biological or not -- what it means to be a family. Within community we learn our roles -- being a wife, husband, mother, father, daughter, son, brother and sister. Most young girls grow up playing with baby dolls while little boys play with trucks, lizards and frogs. Personally, I liked playing with my remote-controlled '57 Chevy. But in the back of my tomboy mind I knew that when I grew up I would be a mommy.

I still have my first baby doll. She has a pretty little porcelain face with peachy cheeks and rosebud lips. Her eyes are sky blue with long brown eye lashes. Her golden blonde hair has ringlet curls tucked under a soft cotton bonnet. Her flowing white Christening gown with delicate eyelet trim has a pretty silk ribbon woven around the waistline. She's the perfect little baby doll. When I wasn't throwing mud at my brother down at the creek, I played with her as a young girl. I imagined having my own 'real' baby one day. I practiced rocking my doll, changing her diapers and feeding her as I spent long lazy hours romanticizing the idea of motherhood.

I remember my mom and grandmother saying, "Honey, when you get old enough you'll meet a wonderful man, get married and have lots of babies." I looked up to them, watching and learning from their examples. I looked forward to the day when my turn would come.

Meeting My Husband

It may not have been as exotic as mom's belly dancing, but I met the man of my dreams in a swing-dance class. He was so very tall, with piercing blue eyes. I experienced the proverbial "pools" and dreamed of swimming in them, actually skinny-dipping. He was amazingly handsome and, to my delight, instantly adored me.

Two years later we tied the knot. Passionate about our new life together, we planned to travel the world living carefree and footloose. We agreed to wait a few years before having children because we knew babies meant sleep deprivation. We also were not ready to be tied down by feeding routines and diaper changes.

"When are you going to start having children?" our parents kept asking.

"When we get ready," Brian and I always replied.

"Well, you're not getting any younger you know," they ever-so-gently reminded us.

Brian and I thought we had all the time in the world and

expected to have two or three children eventually.

> *During a ski trip to Colorado, Lesley and I were having a great week, with perfect snow conditions. While snowboarding one day, I remember seeing a father and his son, about 10 years old, at the bottom of a run. They were obviously having a great time together.*
>
> *The father watched as the boy went over a small jump and nailed the landing. He yelled out, "You rock!"*
>
> *Looking up at his father, the boy said, "No Dad, YOU rock!"*
>
> *As I watched the father and son I thought to myself: One day I'll have my own son and I'll teach him how to snowboard. I'll teach him how to play baseball and surf. Yep, one day....*
>
> **~ Brian**

Controlling Our Reproductive Destiny

Brian and I were determined to enjoy our life as free agents for as long as possible. To prevent pregnancy we used condoms. Unfortunately, they got in the way of spontaneity. We started using coitus interruptus, also known as the pullout, or withdrawal, method. It required no skill or devices and involved no chemicals or artificial hormones. However, the withdrawal method often left us wondering whether we were going to have an "oopsie" baby.

I knew about other methods to prevent pregnancy. But barrier methods, such as the contraceptive sponge, diaphragm, or cervical cap, were not an option for me. The idea of putting a sponge in my vagina was unappealing. Personally, I don't like anything that's not natural.

But, with our growing concern over protecting against having a baby, I reluctantly decided to try probably the most unnatural method—birth control pills. Within three weeks, I gained weight and my emotions were erratic. Poor Brian couldn't say anything without me getting upset. We quickly decided the pill was the culprit, and I dumped what was left in the garbage, swearing never to use anything artificial again.

The only alternative left was Natural Family Planning (NFP), or the rhythm method, used by my Catholic friends. It was simple and cheap. Each morning before getting out of bed, I took my body temperature, and Brian plotted it on a grid to track my highs and lows. Once my temperature spiked, we knew I would soon be fertile, so we refrained from sex during that time. It was a simple method that worked for us.

My Biological Clock

After three fun-filled years of marriage, Brian and I, at 35 and 36 –years old, respectively, decided that it was time to begin our family. Because I've always been healthy, I assumed getting pregnant past the age of 35 would be "no big deal." On a regular basis, I was leg pressing 125 pounds, chest pressing 40 pounds, and able to run three miles while barely breaking a sweat. I was fit as a fiddle and ready for the next phase of our life to begin.

We lived in Pacific Beach (PB), a coastal community in San Diego. PB is like one enormous frat party. All the action takes place on Garnet Avenue, where bars, shops, and clubs line the street. There's a happy hour every day of the week at places like Moondoggies, RT's Longboard Grill, and Lahaina's, and we lived pretty close to the action. During summertime we slept with earplugs to block the noise of neighboring all-night parties. Sunday mornings we ritually cleared our front yard of beer cans and liquor bottles, tossed there by the evening's partygoers.

Because PB was not the kind of environment in which we wanted to raise our children, we sold our condo and bought a four-bedroom house, north of San Diego. It was in a family-oriented community but still close to the beach. Our new community offered topnotch schools, nearby shopping, and convenient work commutes. We were creating the perfect environment for our soon-to-be-expanding family, or so we assumed.

Settled into our new home, we were ready to invite a baby into our world. We were enthusiastic about our baby-making endeavors. We just knew that our incredible love for one another was going to light a fire between one egg and one special sperm to create our little bundle of joy. Every month we held our breath, waiting to see whether or not I was going to start my period.

> *We're trying to conceive and I'm obsessed with baby names. I want to have a name picked out ASAP. Brian thinks we need to get pregnant first. But I'm a planner. I love looking up names on babynamewizard.com, where I can explore naming trends from year to year. If my baby is a boy, I want to name him "Jack" after my grandfather. "Brian Jack" is another possibility and "Christopher Jack" has a nice ring to it. I'm planning for our first baby boy to be born around next February. At least I hope my first kid is a boy. Then we'll have a girl one year later, and another boy two years after that, making a full house. That would be so perfect! Can't wait!*
>
> ~ **Journal, Feb. 6**

High Hopes

After several months of trying to conceive, we questioned why I hadn't gotten pregnant. We were using the rhythm method to track the rising of my body temperature, but something was off. Checking with our doctor we found we had miscalculated the day I was supposed to ovulate. Instead of trying to conceive on days 9 and 11, we needed to have sex on days 12 and 14. At that time we were so green behind our ears that we didn't even know ovulation tests existed.

Finally, I suspected that I was pregnant because I missed my period and my breasts were tender. My nipples hurt so bad that I didn't even want to wear a bra. I considered duct-taping my nipples down but figured Brian would think I was being kinky. Until I was certain of my pregnancy, I didn't want to tell him. I knew something was happening when I started waking up at 5 o'clock in the morning. With an insane rush of energy I spent the early mornings cleaning the house, decluttering the garage, washing clothes, and pulling weeds in the yard. I felt like Superwoman. After a week there were no more house chores to conquer, so I finally drove to the store, bought a test kit, and hurried home.

The first test showed two pink lines, but I thought it could be a false positive. I took a second test and got the same results. Still disbelieving, I called the 1-800 number on the back of the box to make sure I was reading the test correctly.

I was a little nervous making the phone call. On the other end of the phone I heard a male voice speaking with a thick accent. I had expected to hear a woman answer. How could I talk about my urine test with a man? I thought to myself. He doesn't know anything about being pregnant. Then I remembered that he was probably reading from a Q&A script anyway. Eager to know if I performed the test accurately, I spoke hurriedly.

"Hi, I just took the early pregnancy test and I'm not sure if I did it right."

"Well, if you only see one line then you are not pregnant. But if you see two pink lines, then you are pregnant. One line may be lighter than the other. Do you see two lines?"

"Yes, I definitely see two lines. But how pink is pink supposed to be?"

"Well, you should see a solid pink on the first line and the second line should almost match the first pink line."

"Well, my second line is pink, but is it supposed to be pale pink, salmon pink, or more like a fuchsia pink?"

"It really doesn't matter the shade of pink. You can be assured that you are pregnant as long as you see two pink lines. We recommend that you schedule an appointment with your doctor as soon as possible for a full exam and, by the way… congratulations!"

I was so excited. I felt as if my dreams were being realized. After losing my paternal grandparents the previous year, I experienced deep depression and grief. My pregnancy meant new life, a new baby who would bring joy and hope into our lives. I put a lot of expectation into my pregnancy. I felt as if my purpose in life was quickly expanding. I was going to be responsible for bringing another life into the world, caring for my baby, and raising him or her to be a loving person.

Telling Brian

I couldn't wait to tell Brian that I was pregnant, but I wanted to surprise him. I stuffed my positive pregnancy test inside a box of toothpaste and glued it shut. Then, I took the box to Brian and asked for his help to open it. I pretended to be helpless and he bought my act. I could barely stand the anticipation as he worked to pry the small cardboard pieces apart. Maybe I put too much glue on the box, I thought. Finally, he opened it up and pulled out the pregnancy test. The look on his face was priceless: confused because there was no tube of toothpaste; surprised to find a pregnancy test; and excited when he saw the double pink lines.

"You're pregnant?"

"Yes, Honey. I'm pregnant! Can you believe it?"

Brian pulled me into his arms and said, "This is wonderful!"

Spreading Our Good News

As an excited mother-to-be, expecting a healthy pregnancy, I started the nesting process by clearing out the spare bedroom so it could become our baby's room. Brian and I talked about keeping our news confidential until the second trimester, but we could hardly contain ourselves. We were optimistic about the pregnancy and decided to tell family and friends, both to share our joy and gain their emotional support. Being pregnant was new to me and I really wanted to enjoy every moment. To surprise my mom and brother I bought a "Foxy Grandma" T-shirt and a "Best Uncle in the World" trucker's cap. They were totally thrilled.

As the weeks passed we got bolder, telling more and more people. I called my friend in Australia to tell him Lesley was pregnant.

He asked, "Oh, how far along is she?"

"She's in the first trimester."

"Well, it's kinda early and you're already telling people?"

"Oh, we're not worrying about that stuff. We're just telling everybody."

~ Brian

The Roller Coaster

During the first couple of weeks of my pregnancy I felt exceptionally good, almost high. I experienced a bit of spotting but my doctor said it was normal. With Dr. King's permission, I painted our master bedroom a deep terra cotta, keeping the windows open to dispatch paint fumes. As the pregnancy progressed I had days of exhaustion. I still tried to accomplish everything on my to-do list but quickly learned that my pregnant body had limits. Some days, all I could do was lie on the sofa and channel surf, only getting up to urinate or grab something to eat. I was lucky to work from home as a public relations consultant with a flexible work schedule.

> *Brian and I are excited about this pregnancy, though at times it feels like a roller coaster. At week five, Dr. King said my hormone levels hadn't jumped three times as high, as she had expected. So, I did another blood test today. We get results tomorrow. She questioned me about cramps, but I haven't had any. I think everything is fine. It's been a happy-hormone day.*
>
> **~ Journal, April 12**

> *Good news! Dr. King said my hormone levels are now doing great, doubling from day to day. I'm in week six of my pregnancy.*
>
> **~ Journal, April 19**

Week Seven

During week seven, Brian and I went to our first ultrasound appointment at Dr. King's office. First, allow me to say that there is nothing sexy about transvaginal ultrasounds. Imagine lying on an exam table with a plastic banana-like device up your vagina. Not fun. It's very invasive and uncomfortable. The doctor pokes around with the wand until she gets a good display on the monitor, showing the ovaries, fallopian tubes, and uterus. The only benefit is that the device can take photos of the baby, so you can show your family and friends.

As I viewed the ultrasound, I had no idea what I was looking at. The hazy picture was in black and white. Dr. King pointed out my uterus on the monitor.

"Here's your uterus but I don't see a fetus," Dr. King said.

"So, what's that black spot in my uterus? Isn't that my baby?"

"I'm not sure. It's either abnormal development or we have miscounted the number of weeks since conception. But I can't see an embryo. If you are at week seven, then we should be able to see a fetus. Maybe we've miscalculated the days. Maybe you're really at week five, then it's understandable that we're not seeing more on the screen. Let's do another ultrasound in a week. Then we'll know for sure. The fetus will be much easier to see in another week."

> *I'm terrified. I'm living in fear wondering whether or not my baby is growing. I know Brian is scared. I've seen photos of fetuses at week seven. My ultrasound didn't look like the pictures.*
> **~ Journal, April 26**

> *For the next several days I tried not to think about Lesley's ultrasound. I focused on work and went about my routine. I tried not to think about it because there was nothing I could do about it. I tried to ignore the whole thing but wondered if we were headed for a loss instead of a happy ending.*
> **~ Brian**

Nights of Pain

On Thursday night I woke up around 11 o'clock with severe cramps. I thought I needed to go to the bathroom. I tried to get out of bed but, as soon as my feet hit the floor, I collapsed with overwhelming pain. I had no clue what was happening. According to my calendar I was eight weeks pregnant. Brian didn't know what to do. I was in so much agony that I tried to breathe my way through the pain, hoping it would end soon. About 15 minutes later the pain stopped as quickly as it had started. With what little strength I had left, I crawled into bed, feeling exhausted. I fell asleep, thinking I must have eaten something that fiercely disagreed with me.

Two days later, on Saturday afternoon, Brian went to Coachella, a music festival in the desert about three hours from our house. At midnight I awoke with another case of abdominal pain, but this time it was ten times worse. I knew I needed to call for help, but we didn't have a phone in our bedroom and I'd left my cell downstairs. The closest phone was down the hall in the office. I fell to the floor as I tried to get out of bed. The pain was so excruciating that it took my breath away. I couldn't speak. I couldn't yell. I couldn't move. I laid on the floor thinking I was going to die. Time passed and the pain wasn't going away like before. I didn't know what was wrong. I seriously thought that I was dying right then and there. I had never felt so alone in my entire life. Brian was gone and wouldn't be home until Sunday afternoon. I couldn't call for help. I was frozen in agony.

After an hour, the pain lessened a little and I pulled myself up and back into bed. My energy was zapped, my legs were weak, and I felt sick to my stomach. I soon fell asleep. Around 4 a.m. I woke up and walked to the office to call Brian, but his cell phone went straight to voicemail. I told him to come home as soon as possible, and I went back to bed.

To this day I still feel bad about leaving Lesley on Saturday and going to Coachella. I was gone and in a place that didn't have cell phone service. Lesley had more abdominal pain that night. If I had been there, I would have taken her to the emergency room, but she couldn't call anybody. She was basically stuck.

~ Brian

Sunday morning I called my doctor's office.

"Lesley, if you have any more abdominal pain or a bloody discharge, then I want you to go to the emergency room immediately. I'm scheduling you for an ultrasound on Monday morning first thing. Be at our office by 8 o'clock."

On Monday Brian drove me to the doctor's office. We didn't know what to expect.

"Does this hurt? Does this hurt here? Does that hurt?" Dr. King kept asking me as she performed a pelvic exam, pushing around my lower abdomen.

"It's uncomfortable because you're applying a lot of pressure. But it doesn't hurt."

"Well, it should hurt based on what you've told me," Dr. King said with a concerned expression. "We need to do another vaginal ultrasound. Then, we'll run blood tests to measure the levels of your human chorionic gonadotropin (hCG). This is a pregnancy hormone created by the developing embryo and the placenta after conception. If your levels of hCG are low then you could be having an ectopic pregnancy."

What's an Ectopic Pregnancy?

I laid back on the exam table and my doctor inserted the wand-like device into my vagina. Pointing to the ultrasound picture, she shared more information.

"Lesley, this is your uterus. According to your hormone levels, your pregnancy is 7 1/2 to 8 weeks along, and we should be able to see a fetus about the size of a walnut. Unfortunately, I only see this black spot in your uterus, which is either an abnormally developed fetus or could be dried blood. If the spot we're seeing is dried blood, then you may be having an ectopic pregnancy, which means the fetus has implanted itself outside of the uterus. Even though the fetus isn't in your uterus, it will still continue to grow. It's probably in your fallopian tubes, but it can't result in a healthy pregnancy. Unfortunately, the ultrasound is not giving us a good picture of your fallopian tubes."

My mind began to swim in disbelief and confusion. I wondered if the doctor and nurses were conspiring against me. Maybe they were playing a sick joke on me and didn't want me to have a baby. Maybe they randomly choose one pregnant woman each month as the recipient of bad news just like random searches at the airport. It didn't make sense. *How could I be having an ectopic pregnancy when I had always been so healthy?* My doctor didn't have definitive answers for me and I was scared.

"Dr. King, why can't you just take my pregnancy out of the tube and put it into my uterus?"

"I'm sorry, Lesley, but the fetus isn't developing properly in your fallopian tube. There's no way it could survive."

I kept wondering, How do they know the fetus isn't normal? Maybe it's just fine. How can they possibly know the fetus isn't developing if they can't even tell me why it happened? None of it made sense. I was hormonal and emotional, but I finally decided to trust my doctor and hold my crazy thoughts at bay.

Over the past four weeks Brian and I had been looking online at photos of fetal development. We found tons of pictures showing the progression of a baby's development. We had been counting down the days until week seven, when we knew our baby would finally be about the size of a walnut. We knew that the legs would be developing, looking more like little fins than legs, and that the baby's hands would slowly begin to form. It was exciting to imagine that a small fetus would become a big, round, fleshy, bouncing baby in about eight more months. I never realized that the baby's brain and spinal cord began growing as early as seven weeks in a pregnancy. Our baby's heart and lungs would also start to develop along with the eyes, nostrils, and intestines at seven weeks. Brian and I imagined our fetus going through the developmental stages, growing into a little baby—our baby.

Needless to say, this information was in the back of my brain as I laid upon the doctor's exam table.

Dilation and Curettage (D&C)

My blood test confirmed that my hCG hormone level was extremely low.

Dr. King's words brought me back to reality, "I think we need to schedule a dilation and curettage to determine what has happened with your pregnancy. You've either had a miscarriage or you're having an ectopic pregnancy. If we find dried blood in your uterus, then we will know for sure that you are having an ectopic pregnancy. If that's the case, I'll immediately perform a laparoscopy. Your pregnancy is about the size of a walnut and it will burst your fallopian tube soon if left untreated. It could be fatal if you can't get to an emergency room. If caught earlier, an injection of methotrexate would dissolve the pregnancy but it's too late for that option now. There isn't time for it to take effect. I want to schedule your surgery for the day after tomorrow."

The words dilation and curettage sent up red flags in my mind. I knew what that meant. D&C, the common name for a dilation and curettage, can also be the code for an abortion. Having grown up in Mississippi, I remembered hearing Bible-thumping ministers preach against abortion. I wondered if those same preachers would call me a sinner for having a medically necessary D&C.

The situation was out of my control and my life was at stake. Dr. King was worried that my fallopian tube would burst causing internal bleeding. The fetus inside my fallopian tube never had a heartbeat as it couldn't develop normally. I trusted Dr. King and felt confident she would take care of me. Everything was happening so fast that I didn't have a lot of time to dwell on things.

How Do You Pronounce Laparoscopy?

"Dr. King, I know what a D&C is but what is a laparoscopy? It sounds awful."

"Laparoscopy is actually not as bad as it sounds. It's minimally invasive surgery. I'll be making three small incisions in your abdominal area, one through your belly button and one on each side of your hips near your bikini line. We'll inflate your abdomen with carbon dioxide gas to enable us to see and get to your fallopian tubes and ovaries. Then I'll insert a laparoscope, a small telescope with a light and camera, letting us see what's going on in your abdomen. Once we confirm that your pregnancy is in your tubes, then we'll remove it. You'll be under anesthesia during the procedure so you won't feel a thing. The benefit of us doing the laparoscopy is that I'll be able to evaluate your ovaries and tubes, check for any other issues and inspect your uterus. It's an outpatient procedure. So, after you wake up and feel good enough you'll be able to go home."

Great, I'll be able to go home, I sarcastically thought to myself. I was pissed, actually angry, that this was happening to me. I felt like my body was being disloyal to me. I have always tried to take care of myself: never smoked, never took drugs, ate healthy and exercised regularly. Now, none of my efforts made a difference. It wasn't fair and didn't make sense.

Brian and I left the doctor's office feeling like someone had stolen our dreams. Sadness engulfed our hearts. We felt helpless.

On Wednesday morning we were sick at heart, knowing our baby would never be born. We drove to the hospital in silence. A nurse led me to a little room where I took off my clothes and stuffed them into a metal locker. After I put the hospital gown on, the nurse asked me questions about pain management.

"On a scale of 1 to 10, one being the least and ten being the greatest, how much pain do you want to feel?"

"Are you serious? I don't want to feel a thing. Zero pain. Drug me up," I said boldly thinking that was the one thing I could control. "I'm in enough emotional pain as it is, and don't see any reason to go through physical pain."

The nurse escorted Brian and me into the pre-op room. We

were greeted by the anesthesiologist who tried to be funny, "What kind of cocktail would you like today?"

"I would like a mango martini—and make it strong," I said with as much of a smile as I could muster.

A few minutes later Dr. King walked into the room and I started crying. Her presence affirmed the fact that I was about to lose my baby. I felt a little panicky. "Can you tell us why you are here today?" she asked.

Trying not to completely fall apart I explained, "I'm here today because I've either miscarried or I'm having an ectopic pregnancy. We're not sure which one yet. You're going to do a D&C procedure to determine if my pregnancy is a miscarriage or if I'm having an ectopic. Because we can't see a fetus in my uterus, we know something is wrong with my pregnancy. You said that you will review the blood from my uterus under a microscope. If it's not pregnancy material and just dried blood, then you'll know I have an ectopic, at which point you will perform a laparoscopy to remove my pregnancy from my fallopian tube. I think that's about it from what I understand."

Tears streamed down my face. The anesthesiologist gave me the mango martini which helped me relax a bit. I sat looking around the room, waiting.

"I'm still awake. That mango martini isn't strong enough. You might want to hit me again," I informed the anesthesiologist.

Brian leaned over and gave me a kiss saying, "It's all going to be all right."

Next thing I knew the lights went out.

Waking Up

Excruciating pain ripped through my lower abdomen. I wanted to yell, "I'm in pain," but the words coming out of my mouth were unrecognizable. My eyes wouldn't open. The anesthesia kept me groggy.

Vomit projected from my esophagus. Someone turned my head to the side and held a container up to my chin. My arms wouldn't move. I felt helpless. The person wiped my mouth with a wet washcloth. I wondered if the stranger had superglued my eyes shut.

Time passed. I muttered the only words I could summon to my lips, "I'm in pain."

A female voice said, "You're supposed to be in pain. You just got out of surgery."

That comment cut right to my heart. I was pissed and cussed her in my mind. You bitch! How dare you say that to me! Do you even realize that I just lost my baby? Oh, if I could talk, I'd give you a piece of my mind.

I was out of my mind with pain. And helpless. It wasn't a good feeling. I wanted to throw something at her. I wanted to scream for her manager. But all I could mumble was, "I'm in pain. I'm in pain. I'm in pain."

More time passed and my eyes opened to see the sarcastic culprit who wouldn't give me drugs.

"Where is my husband? I want to see my husband," I informed her.

"We'll call him after you're more awake."

Finally, Dr. King appeared out of nowhere, "How are you feeling, Lesley?"

"Horrible. I'm in excruciating pain and I want drugs," I said definitively.

"Okay, we'll get you started on morphine. But first, let me check you out."

Dr. King pushed down on my abdomen, "Does this hurt?"

"Hell yes that hurts!"

"Okay, good. After the surgery you just had, it should hurt," Dr. King said with a smile. "Your surgery went very well. When I did the D&C, there was no pregnancy material in your uterus. There was only dried blood as I suspected. At that point I knew you had an ectopic pregnancy so I performed a laparoscopy. The pregnancy was in your left fallopian tube. So, I made a small incision in your left tube to remove the pregnancy but I didn't remove any of your tube. Your ovaries and internal organs looked really healthy. I can tell that you've never smoked. You had a lot of internal bleeding because your fallopian tube had already started to burst. I can't believe that you weren't in more pain. You are a tough cookie. As much internal bleeding as you were having you should have been in major pain over the last 24 hours."

"Well, tell my husband that I'm a tough cookie because he thinks I'm a wimp. Now, will you pump me up with morphine? And will you please tell the nurse to get my husband in here?"

"Sure," Dr. King said.

I could see the concern on Brian's face when he walked into the room. "Honey, how are you doing? I've been worried. Your surgery took a lot longer than I had expected."

"I'm okay now that you're here. Dr. King has something to tell you."

Recovery

Although I was supposed to be released as an outpatient, Dr. King suggested I stay overnight at the hospital. My pain wasn't going away and I didn't feel good enough to walk. They put me on the maternity floor in a private room that had been decorated for a newborn baby and mother. Once I was settled, Brian left the hospital to go home and walk Baby, our Bichon Frise, who had been cooped up all afternoon and evening.

Two nurses were in and out of my room every few minutes. One nurse had short red hair with cute freckles dotting her nose and cheeks. The other nurse was a soft spoken brunette with a smile that lit up the room.

Around 11 o'clock that night I needed to urinate.

"I really need to go to the bathroom but I'm not sure I can walk and I'm hurting so badly in my abdomen that I'm scared to pee," I said feeling a little embarrassed.

"It's okay honey, we'll take care of you. That's what we're here for," the red head said.

They walked me to the bathroom. I felt nauseous and dizzy as

35

if I would pass out. Turning around I sat down on the commode. The brunette stood next to me, holding me up. She placed a cold rag on my forehead. I could see the other nurse heating up another wash cloth which she placed on my stomach to relax my muscles. I was getting royal treatment.

"I'm hurting so bad. If I pee will my stitches rip out or will I start bleeding?"

"No, you'll be okay. Just take your time and breathe. Try to relax." She turned the faucet on and let the water run. Then, she started singing to me.

Finally, I relaxed. It felt so good to empty my bladder. My insides didn't fall out and it took the pressure off of my uterus.

The nurses tucked me back into bed and brought me Italian ice. "Honey, this won't make you sick. You need to get something into your stomach since you haven't had anything to eat all day."

The Italian ice tasted wonderfully sweet going down my throat. I had the best nurses in the world. I never wanted to leave. Brian came back around midnight and slept on the cot beside my bed.

The next morning a new nurse appeared in my room. She seemed anxious to get me moving and walking around so I could go home. Little did she know, I didn't really want to leave. Once I got home I doubted I would receive five-star treatment. Brian would do the best he could, but there'd be no Italian ice cream.

When it was time to leave, Brian helped me into a wheelchair and pushed me down the hallway. The walls were painted in soft pinks and pastel blues. Baby photos lined the desk at the nurses' station. The women smiled and waved goodbye to me. Do they think I had a baby or do they know about my loss, I wondered. Guess it doesn't matter. I'll never see them again.

I left the maternity ward with no baby, just stitches, a lot of pain and a bottle of Vicodin. My heart ached as much as my abdomen. I popped a morphine pill wishing it would numb my mind. I wanted my thoughts to stop. Brian and I felt sad because our dream of starting our own little family had been surgically removed. We felt hopeless not knowing whether I would ever get pregnant again.

Our desire to have a child together was rooted in our affection and commitment to one another. Brian thought it would be cute to have a little Lesley running around. I wanted two or three kids and grandchildren one day. I pictured big holiday gatherings as a matriarch, but first I had to have a baby.

As Brian drove me home, I thought about taking the entire bottle of Vicodin but had enough sense to know that would be stupid. I felt like someone had tossed my heart into the ocean without a lifeline. Would I sink or swim? Only time would tell.

Having experienced grief from the loss of my grandparents, I knew time was the only thing that would help me. In time I would forget the physical pain. In time my scars would fade. In time I would laugh again. But knowing that didn't help much. I decided to take things minute by minute, and be thankful I was alive and grateful for my loving husband.

My feeble attempt at optimism was a mask to hide my depression from myself. I hated what was happening. I wanted to scream at the universe for not getting what I wanted, but screaming wouldn't change anything. I had absolutely no control. That's what really freaked me out. My action, inaction, thoughts, prayers, or lack thereof seemed to make no difference. Brian and I didn't say much on the drive home. We just held hands.

For the next three days Brian took care of me around the clock. My stomach muscles were so sore that I needed help just standing up and sitting down. I religiously took Vicodin to ward off most of the pain. When Brian was at work, my mother-in-law graciously sat with me. She prepared my meals and even searched high and low for Italian ice at three grocery stores. When she couldn't find it, she surprised me with mango, raspberry, and lemon sorbets, which were equally delicious. She proved an even better caregiver than the hospital nurses.

Following my laparoscopic procedure, I endured endless blood tests. Dr. King wanted to make sure my hCG pregnancy hormone returned to zero. Visiting the lab each week was a constant reminder of the baby I had lost. I cried every time they drew my blood. The needle didn't hurt, but my heart was in pain. I was devastated and felt like a complete failure.

After the laparoscopy and D&C procedures, Dr. King informed me that my body needed to heal from the surgery. "Chances are you'll have a miscarriage if you get pregnant within the next three months."

> *Lesley was in a lot of pain after the laparoscopy and D&C. The doctor only made three small incisions for the laparoscopy, but it was not a "jog home from the hospital" type of surgery. Lesley was laid up in bed and couldn't even move the first day. She was on morphine. It took a while for the pain to go away. For weeks after her surgery, I didn't want us to have sex because I was scared it was too soon and I'd hurt her. I also didn't want to get her pregnant too soon. Her body wasn't ready to carry a baby and needed to heal. My top priority was getting her well.*
>
> **~ Brian**

Over the next few weeks, I became a recluse and fell into deep depression. I ignored friends by not returning phone calls and even quit playing tennis. All I wanted to do was sit on the sofa and stare at the TV to escape my life. I was emotionally stressed and traumatized. It was frightening to think about how close I came to death without even realizing that something was seriously wrong with me. I found out the hard way that an ectopic is the leading cause (10 percent) of pregnancy-related deaths. I never envisioned that being pregnant could be so complicated.

Hysterosalpingogram (HSG)

Brian and I worried about whether or not I'd be able to get pregnant again. Dr. King said I had a 10 to 20 percent chance of having a second ectopic, depending on the condition of my tubes. So she suggested that I undergo a hysterosalpingogram (HSG), which is used to determine if either or both of the fallopian tubes are open or blocked. (The tubes should be open and connected to the uterus, so the sperm can travel up the tubes to meet and fertilize an egg.)

Dr. King promised that the test would be quick and painless. No big deal. So, I made an appointment, assuming it would give me peace of mind to know what was going on inside my reproductive system.

Well, if you really want to know how tough you are, then have an HSG. I wouldn't wish the test on my worst enemy, especially if she had a blocked tube.

I remember walking into the surgical room for my procedure. The room was very sterile looking. White walls. White flooring. White linens. Tons of stainless steel equipment everywhere. Large flat-screen TV monitors hung on every wall as if it were a sports bar. Computers lined the desk next to the patient table. It was intimidating.

The nurse told me to undress from my waist down and then stepped out of the room. Brian folded my clothes and placed them on a nearby chair. I climbed onto the futuristic stainless steel table, sinking heavily into the three-inch foam mattress, and draped the thin white sheet over me.

"I'm glad that I don't have to lie butt naked on this hard, cold table. That would be miserable, but I guess not as miserable as what the doctor is about to do to me."

"Well, this test is important," Brian assured me. "It's going to give us more information, so we know what to do next. I don't want you having another ectopic pregnancy. I don't want to take that risk. It's too dangerous."

"Well, now that I've had one ectopic, I'm not worried about having another one. Dr. King said they would be screening me earlier throughout my next pregnancy since I'm high risk. If I did have another ectopic, they would at least catch it earlier than the first one."

"I'm serious. I don't want to take the chance."

"Well, how do you expect us to have a baby and not run the risk of having another ectopic pregnancy?"

"We could do IVF. I think they just bypass your tubes and implant the embryo in your uterus. You don't even have to worry about the whole ectopic issue."

"Oh, no. I don't think so. It's way too expensive, and all those needles. Do you really want me to suffer a billion needles in my butt? We know I can get pregnant. It was just a fluke that my first pregnancy turned out to be a tubal pregnancy. It probably won't happen again. I'd rather try getting pregnant on my own and run the small risk of having another ectopic than do IVF treatments. At least I know what to expect with an ectopic. I've been through it once. I've heard horror stories from friends who have done IVF. I'm not doing it. No way."

"Well, I don't want you to be stuck somewhere bleeding to death from an ectopic, with me not there to help you."

"You're worrying for nothing. That's not going to happen."

The radiologist knocked on the door. Entering the room, she shook our hands and gave me a quick overview of the HSG procedure.

"We are going to take an x-ray of your uterus and fallopian tubes today. Using a long, small tube, I will inject blue dye through your cervix into the uterus and tubes. The dye allows me to see if there is blockage or any other problem. All you have to do is remain still. We want to get the best possible picture for you. Are you ready to begin?"

"Sure."

Brian took his place standing next to my head, where he had a great view of the monitor showing my insides. Ceiling tiles filled my line of vision.

The radiologist guided my feet to the stirrups and asked me to scoot closer to the edge of the table.

"Okay, here we go. First, I'm inserting a speculum into your vagina, just like your doctor does during a pap smear. This will allow me to see your cervix. Next, I'm inserting a thin catheter through your cervix and into your uterus. You might feel a slight pinch when it goes through your cervix. Are you okay?"

"It's a little uncomfortable but I'm okay."

"Now, I'm releasing the dye through the catheter into your uterus. We'll be able to see the size and shape of your uterus. When your uterus fills up, the dye will flow into your fallopian tubes, and we should see the dye spilling out the other side of your tubes into your abdominal cavity."

"What happens to the dye then?"

"It gets reabsorbed by your body. It won't hurt you. The dye is flowing through your right fallopian tube. So, that one is open and clear, but there's a blockage in your left tube. Didn't you say you had an ectopic?"

"Yes, in my left tube. My OB-GYN did a laparoscopy. She said there might be scar tissue left over."

"There's definite blockage. I'm going to try and force the dye through your left tube. Sometimes forcing dye through the tube will dislodge any material that's blocking it. This will probably be uncomfortable. Are you ready?"

"Yes."

I felt pressure in my lower abdomen at first but, as she tried to force dye through my tube, it felt like menstrual cramps. Then, a moment later, I experienced excruciating abdominal pain, making it hard to breathe. I grabbed Brian's hand and squeezed. I kept thinking it wasn't going to last long.

"How are you doing?"

"Not good. How much longer?"

My high threshold for pain dissolved. Tears streamed down my face, but I laid perfectly still, waiting for the torture to end.

"Just give me a couple more minutes. I'm trying my best to dislodge the blockage in your tube. Hang in there."

The agony overwhelmed me. I put a death grip on the table and screamed, "It hurts! It hurts! Oh God it hurts."

Brian bent down to get closer to me and looked straight into my eyes. Stroking my hair he said, "Honey, look at me. I want you to focus on me."

He held my hand and kept stroking my hair.

"It's okay. You're going to be okay. It's almost over. She's just about done. Hang in there. This will help. We're going to know what's going on. I'm here, honey. I'm right here. Squeeze my hand as hard as you need to."

I squeezed Brian's hand with all my strength. Tears poured down my cheeks and I gasped between each breath. After a few more minutes the radiologist finally gave up.

"I'm sorry. I wasn't able to dislodge the blockage, but at least we know your right tube is open."

I said nothing. I was thankful it was over.

The Journey
Coping
In the bright morning light
Praying
Asking for joy to make it right
Failing
My heart and thoughts blur
Needing
Hope to help me endure
Seeking
A pathway right and pure
Knowing
Peace will soon be mine
Waiting
For Love's touch so divine
—Lesley Vance

Clearing Up Misconceptions

Couples are considered infertile if they have not been able to get pregnant within 12 months of having frequent, unprotected sex.[1] No one likes to admit to being infertile but, by definition, it is a medical condition. There are physiological reasons why men and women experience infertility. Again, infertility is a medical condition. The most common causes of infertility include blocked fallopian tubes, poor ovulation, endometriosis, polycystic ovarian syndrome (a hormone disorder that causes cysts on the ovaries), low sperm count, poor sperm motility, and poor sperm morphology. Infertility is not something that you can just get over by "relaxing" and "going on a vacation."

More about Ectopics: Blocked Fallopian Tubes

Blocked fallopian tubes cause ectopic, or tubal, pregnancies and are the cause of fertility problems in 40 percent of infertile women. The word "ectopic" comes from the Greek word ektopos and literally means "out of place." Of every 50 pregnancies, 1 is "out of place," meaning the pregnancy is not in the uterus. Of those women having ectopic pregnancies, 10 to 15 percent will never be able to have children. For the most part, the cause of tubal pregnancies is unknown. Suspected culprits may be sexually transmitted infections in the uterus, tubes, or ovaries, which can cause scarring. Other causes include:
- fallopian tube damage from previous surgeries or scarring
- endometriosis (the presence of the uterine lining outside the uterus, such as on the ovaries)
- aging
- smoking nicotine
- fertility drugs

How Do You Know if You Have an Ectopic?

The symptoms are not always obvious; it depends on your threshold for pain. With an ectopic, you may or may not have early signs of pregnancy, such as sore breasts, spot bleeding, and nausea. Everyone is different. Some women have a brownish discharge one week or so after missing their period. They assume the discharge is their normal menstrual cycle. I experienced episodes of severe abdominal pain, dizziness, spotting, and nausea. If I hadn't contacted my doctor, I would have ended up in the emergency room at best. So, it's important to take your situation seriously. Call your doctor if you have any signs of a potential ectopic pregnancy. Don't second-guess yourself or minimize your experience.

History of Ectopics

Sometimes we forget about the past and take our medical advances for granted. Today we have a lot of knowledge about ectopic pregnancies: signs, symptoms, treatments, and preventive care. I thought I had it rough with my first ectopic, but hundreds of thousands of women have died in previous generations because they didn't have the luxury of modern technology.

Doctors first documented an ectopic pregnancy in the 11th century. Since the beginning of time, most ectopic pregnancies have resulted in the woman's death. In 1759, the first successful operation was performed to treat an ectopic pregnancy. Still, only 1 in 6 women survived the early primitive-type of operation. Surprisingly, the survival rate for women not receiving surgery was actually better: one out of three.

Finally, in the 20th century, medical improvements were introduced, including anesthesia, antibiotics, and blood transfusions. These breakthroughs gave women a fighting chance when faced with a compromised pregnancy. In 1970, the Centers for Disease Control and Prevention (CDC) began documenting the occurrences of ectopic pregnancies in women, reporting 17,800 cases.[2] Medical advancements have continued to save more and more women's lives, and the CDC has progressed in its ability to collect data, giving us more reliable information.[2] Today in the United States, 3.2 percent of all pregnancy losses are ectopics. That's about 64,000 women who experience tubal pregnancy loss each year.[3]

when things go wrong

We live in a culture that teaches us to expect certain outcomes at certain times in our lives. It's no wonder we end up experiencing grave disappointments when things go wrong, leaving us bitter and angry.

Let's Be Honest

No one wants to hear about pregnancies that go wrong. Most people don't want to think about fetuses that die at nine, fifteen or twenty-four weeks of gestation. They certainly don't want to talk about the gory details of ectopics and miscarriages. It's depressing. Conversations about laparoscopies and D&Cs remind us that things don't always work out.

After my pregnancy loss, I read various infertility websites and medical journals. I was surprised to learn that 2 million pregnancies end in loss each year in the United States, and 7.3 million women ages 15 - 44 experience infertility problems.[1, 3] I bet these women probably feel a lot like me. It's as if we all got dropped during Rush Week, with little hope of receiving membership into the Mommy Sorority.

Because pregnancy loss is not often talked about outside a doctor's office, many women are afraid to say "I lost my baby," "I had a miscarriage and my baby died at 14 weeks," or "My baby was growing outside of my uterus and there was no way for it to survive." Men are even less encouraged to talk about their feelings regarding infertility challenges. When you're in the midst of it, pregnancy loss and infertility are very painful if not impossible to discuss.

Baby Showers

I absolutely despise going to baby showers, but it's not because I'm jealous of the pregnant mother unwrapping a hundred gifts. I wish to avoid all the personal questions that women I've never met before invariably ask.

The worst knife to the heart? "How many children do you have?" This question feels like the woman standing before me is a completely self-absorbed idiot. Can't she see my pain? Granted, she may or may not be a self-absorbed idiot. It's possible that she is just trying to connect with me and make conversation. Nevertheless, the question assumes that my world is "normal" and I have a truckload of babies waiting for me at home. Obviously, she has children and why wouldn't I too? Why? In this situation, I usually excuse myself and seek out a tall glass of champagne to calm my nerves. The truth is that her question cuts right to the quick. I grieve all over again.

Another popular question is, "Do you have children?" At least the woman asking this question isn't making an assumption. She gets credit for that, but I still dislike the question because it reminds me that I feel like a complete failure when it comes to making babies. Most of the time I just say, "No, I don't have children," and change the subject.

Unfortunately, some women don't take the hint. They ask, "Why don't you have children? Don't you want children?" It feels like the women asking this question are looking at me like I'm a freak and that something is wrong with me. The question makes me physically flinch with pain. My tears surface when I hear it.

Maybe I should reply, "Well, actually I want children, but this is a difficult subject for me to talk about because I've had pregnancy problems."

I don't share that information because I know from trial and error that it only opens a can of worms. Often women suggest that I adopt or use donor eggs, doling out advice as if they have the perfect answer for me.

Before my losses, I also thought that if you wanted babies you would have them. So, I understand the questions are not really intended to hurt my feelings. These women are just trying to find common ground. In Chapter 7 I suggest "things to say" and "things not to say" to people you meet at baby showers and other places, like grocery stores, libraries, shopping malls, and parties. It's tough living in a world where most women take motherhood for granted, thinking that everyone has babies. The truth is that sometimes things can go terribly wrong.

Carol and Nick's Story: Miscarriage

Carol and Nick never imagined that they would have problems procreating. They already had two healthy, beautiful children. Carol's pregnancies had been a breeze and her deliveries were uneventful. Because having children seemed so easy and natural for Carol, she wanted to have another baby. When the time was right, she quit taking birth control pills. Two years later, at the age of 39, Carol conceived.

> *I had a little bleeding during the first few weeks of my pregnancy, but my doctor assured us that everything was okay. He said, "Don't worry. Fifty percent of my patients bleed during pregnancy and have healthy babies. It's normal."*
>
> *At the end of my first trimester, I had a blood clot outside of my embryonic sac, meaning that I was having internal bleeding. Yet, the ultrasound showed our baby girl dancing around and progressing at a normal rate. We thought everything was fine.*
>
> *Unfortunately, my mother died of cancer when I was 14 weeks along in my pregnancy. I was crushed by the loss. Wondering where God was in the midst of everything, I prayed, "Please let my baby have blue*

eyes just like my mom's blue eyes, so I will have a reminder of her. I need to know you hear me, God, and that you will answer my prayer."

After mom's funeral I started having the most incredible pain. I thought it was appendicitis, so Nick rushed me to the hospital. Dr. Henry couldn't find a reason for my pain, and our baby seemed fine. It was a complete mystery. During the next month, the same scenario kept happening.

At 19 weeks I woke up knowing something was different. Watching me get out of the shower Nick said, "Your belly looks smaller today."

"Yeah, I think so too. I'll call Dr. Henry for a checkup."

After additional blood tests the doctor said our baby might have spina bifida, a condition in which the baby's spine doesn't close during the first months of pregnancy. He wanted to do an amniocentesis and take a small sample of the amniotic fluid around the baby to rule out certain birth defects and genetic disorders.

Even if something was wrong, I planned on carrying my baby to term.

When Dr. Henry did the amniocentesis, there wasn't enough fluid to withdraw. He injected blue dye into the amniotic sac, and we waited to see if I discharged the blue dye, which would mean there was a tear in the sac.

On the ultrasound we could see that our baby was having an irregular heartbeat. "Is my baby going to suffocate if I lose the amniotic fluid? Is this causing her pain?"

"You have to understand that we just injected a foreign substance into her home. She has to adjust," Dr. Henry explained.

Her heartbeat finally returned to normal.

A few hours passed. I went to the bathroom. As I sat down, blood and blue dye poured out of me, filling the toilet.

Dr. Henry and other neonatal specialists told me that I needed to stay at the hospital on bed rest for the next 10 weeks, until the baby was viable. With a 7- and 10-year-old at home, I didn't know how Nick would be able to take care of them and run his business. I felt overwhelmed, knowing I had to stay at the hospital.

My best friend, Helen, came to the hospital to stay with me. We sent Nick home to be with the kids. Later that night I asked the nurse to let me hear my baby's heartbeat again. She placed the baby monitor on my stomach, but I didn't hear a heartbeat.

"Don't get upset, now. It's an old baby monitor. I'll order an ultrasound," the nurse said.

We saw my baby, but there was no heartbeat on the ultrasound. In order to declare that a baby's dead, they have to perform two ultrasounds, administered by two different doctors. They were going to call another doctor immediately to do the second ultrasound, so they could give me the labor and delivery medicines right away, if needed.

I asked, "What happens if we wait until the morning? Why get the doctor away from his family, if it can wait until the morning?"

Giving me a sleeping pill, the neonatal specialist agreed to wait until the morning.

When Nick arrived, the doctors gave me medication to force my body into labor. They don't do C-sections for stillbirths because there's a high risk of infection.

I waited and waited. After 30 hours of waiting, I

wanted everything to be over.

Wondering about my baby, I asked the nurse if there was any possibility that her eyes would be open when she came out.

"No, there's no way. It's too early in her development for her eyes to be open. At 19 weeks the eyes are dark—almost black. Her eyes will be fused shut and the skin will be thin. She'll be about nine to ten inches long, and her head will be the size of a tennis ball. What you see in the ultrasound photos are distorted. Do you and your husband want us to take care of the baby, or do you want to put the baby in the hospital's cemetery?"

"We're going to have her cremated."

After another six hours my baby came out. It happened quickly. I didn't have to push at all. Nick said he didn't want to be there. I remember him saying, "There is nothing in me that wants to see a dead baby." Dr. Henry told him that I needed him to be with me, whether or not he watched what was happening.

The moment arrived when I finally saw our baby. She was seven ounces and nine to ten inches long. She had ten fingers and ten toes, and when I opened her mouth there was a little bitty tongue. The miracle was that her eyes were open and they were blue, just like my mom's eyes. We named her Audrey.

Seeing her blue eyes was extremely comforting to me. I felt like it was a miracle, as if God was letting me know that he heard my prayer.

The nurse said, "It's amazing that in gestation her eyes were open. That doesn't happen. At 19 weeks babies don't open their eyes."

After the nurses cleaned her up, Nick and I held her. The nurse brought in a little baby ring and an *eyelet dress that would fit a baby doll. She took pictures, saying, "It may be hard for you to look at, but one day you might want to see these photos." The nurse then made her handprints and footprints.*

Our baby was perfectly formed, except for the tiny tear in her stomach where her intestines were coming out. She had an abdominal hernia, which is a genetic disorder. It's a tiny tear in the stomach. Hers never closed and her organs developed outside of her abdomen. It's why she tested so high for spina bifida. I had thirteen ultrasounds in four different hospitals in two different states, and none of the doctors saw the abdominal hernia.

Because of my mom's death, my family and I had envisioned grand plans for this baby. Nick and I heard about another lady in the hospital who had a baby at 21 weeks, and her baby survived. We were so close. We wondered so many times why in the world it happened this way.

When we had our first two children, we were so proud and sent out baby photos to everyone we knew. But with this pregnancy I had nothing to share.

After receiving more than a hundred sympathy cards, we decided to send an announcement telling everyone our baby's weight and giving people a chance to know more about Audrey. We added a photo that showed the bottom of her feet, because we wanted everyone to know she was real. After having our baby cremated, we held a private memorial service and put her ashes in a little urn the size of a salt shaker.

The doctors called my pregnancy a miscarriage because it was at 19 weeks. Any time a fetus dies in the womb during the first 19 weeks, they call it a miscarriage. But if your baby dies at 20 weeks or beyond, then the doctors call it a stillbirth. I felt like my baby was a stillbirth, even if she arrived seven days before the official cut-off date.

After I got out of the hospital I felt lost. I was furious with the word "miscarriage." If you misplace, you have placed something in the wrong place. If you miscalculate, you were wrong in your calculation. So, if you miscarry you carried it wrong. The implication of that word is so wrong. It just ticked me off.

During the next year, I was sure each month that I would be pregnant again. Grief makes you insane. I had never hurt so badly before in my life. And of course it was compounded because I had just lost my mom. I couldn't call my mom on the phone to talk to her about what I was going through. One day I started crying and couldn't stop. I couldn't sleep either. I'd wake up in the middle of the night hearing a baby cry. I finally met with a counselor who specializes in children's death. The most profound thing the doctor said that sticks in my head is that it takes seven years to grieve the loss of a child. We expect our parents to die but not a child.

~ **Carol**

More about Miscarriages

The most ridiculous thing I ever heard my doctor say was, "You have had a normal miscarriage." I would like to know what's normal about having a miscarriage. There's nothing normal about 600,000 women suffering every year in the United States from a miscarriage. About 50 percent of all miscarriages occur within the first 12 weeks of pregnancy due to some type of chromosome abnormality in the embryo (the first eight weeks) or fetus (nine weeks to birth).

Sometimes the egg or sperm cell will have too few or too

many chromosomes (structure of genetic information and protein that's found in cells), making it impossible for a healthy embryo to develop. The body often deals with these dysfunctional embryos by naturally expelling them. Chromosomes are the substance of life itself, containing the necessary blueprint for all organisms to develop and function. Without properly functioning chromosomes, no embryo or fetus will survive and thrive into a healthy live birth.

Other factors can also increase a woman's chance of having a miscarriage,[4] including hormone imbalances, thyroid problems, infections, smoking, maternal trauma, drinking alcohol, using illicit drugs, improper implantation of the embryo into the uterine lining, diabetes, maternal age, and autoimmune disorders such as Hashimoto's thyroiditis.

Lori's Story: Symptoms and Treatments for a Miscarriage

Lori, a thirty-three-year-old woman who had been struggling with infertility for five years, had a hard time detecting her miscarriage, because many of the symptoms occur in a normal pregnancy. Vaginal bleeding, abdominal pain, fatigue, backache, and cramps are all indicators of both. She felt zero symptoms to suggest that she might be having a miscarriage. Her ultrasound proved otherwise. Lori spoke about her treatment options.

> *My doctor said that it would be all right for me to allow my body to naturally expel the pregnancy, but he said it could take up to six weeks. As another option he offered me drugs to speed up the process. My third option was to undergo a D&C to remove the fetus. I didn't feel okay about waiting and not knowing when it was going to happen. I knew that if all of the tissue didn't come out eventually, my doctor would be doing a D&C on me anyway to prevent infection.*
>
> *I didn't really like any of the options, but I decided*

to have a D&C. I was terrified that I would start hemorrhaging while driving 75 miles per hour down the interstate or in line at the grocery store or sitting at my desk at work. The whole thing freaked me out. I wanted to know when my pregnancy was going to end. I wanted some form of control in what I felt like was a very uncontrollable situation. I figured having a D&C was the healthiest way to prepare my womb to heal and get ready for my next pregnancy.

~ **Lori**

Michael and Lisa's Story: Stillbirth

Michael, a thirty-four-year-old general manager in the hospitality industry, and Lisa, a thirty-four-year-old floral designer, got married in 2002. They brought one child each into the relationship from previous marriages. Because of their strong belief in family, Michael and Lisa decided that they really wanted to have a child together. Since they were in their early 30s, it never occurred to them that there could be a problem. Michael shares their story.

Lisa became pregnant right away after we got married. Early on there were no problems. Our doctor did the normal First Trimester Screen, which is a blood test and an ultrasound to identify risk for things like Down Syndrome.

There were no genetic disorders in either side of our families, so we were shocked when the tests showed a potential for Down Syndrome. We knew that it meant that our baby could be mentally retarded, develop slowly, or have other problems. Then we were faced with the decision about whether to do an amnio. We were scared to let the doctor put a needle through Lisa's abdomen and into her uterus to withdraw fluid from the amniotic sac. They use ultrasound to guide the needle and to make sure the fetal heartbeat is normal, but it's still a risk. We did the test anyway, and Lisa's amnio came back absolutely positive.

The doctor asked us to decide if we wanted to continue with Lisa's pregnancy. We didn't know what to do. We were completely confused. I was knee-deep in a brand new job and it was an incredibly stressful time. We decided to put off the decision until we could learn more about Down Syndrome.

A couple of weeks later Lisa had another ultrasound, and we got even worse news. I remember the nurse saying, "Wow, this baby is really sick. Let me get the doctor."

The doctor came into our room, looked at the ultrasound and said, "Lisa and Michael, we've got a different problem here. Fluid is building up around your baby's head and neck. One of three things is going to happen: He'll go into cardiac arrest in the womb, meaning his heart will stop beating and your pregnancy will end in stillbirth; he'll be born with the fluid and he'll have to have surgery to fix that; or it will go away."

Lisa and I did not want to terminate her pregnancy. We were scared to death, but we were hoping for the best. We knew there were different levels of Down Syndrome children. Some are dependent their entire life and others can hold a job.

As it turned out, we didn't have time to make a decision, because our baby went into cardiac arrest and died in Lisa's womb.

It broke my heart when our baby's heartbeat stopped. Lisa's pregnancy had been a breeze during the first 20 weeks. We were devastated that it ended as a stillbirth.

The hardest part was when Lisa had to deliver our baby. Everything happened so fast. They gave her medicine to induce labor and an epidural. It was almost like she was drunk, because she wasn't really sure what was going on. Without even realizing it, she delivered the baby.

The nurse placed our baby on a little table and asked us, "Do you want to see him?"

We said, "No." But before they took him away we changed our minds and said, "Yeah, actually we do."

The nurses wrapped him up and gave him to Lisa. We sat there and looked at him. He was five months old and he looked perfect to us. He was our son. At that point we immediately decided that he needed to be a part of our lives. We had a ceremony, named him Daniel, and got a birth certificate for him. We chose to have him cremated. He's on our mantel at home and part of our family. Every year for his birthday we release balloons in his honor and wish him Happy Birthday. It's a big bawl fest.

I can't even begin to explain all of my emotions. It was very difficult, but we didn't want our baby to be taken and discarded. He was ours. Especially for Lisa and me; he was the first baby that we had together. We just needed him to be a part of us. Having the ceremony and cremation turned out to be the best thing for us.

It was a lot to get over. For months afterward we wondered why it happened. We didn't have any answers and we didn't try to seek any out. I've always believed that things happen for a reason, and if we can't figure out what went wrong in the moment, then it will be shown at some point in the future.

Maybe we took our 18- and 12-year-old sons for

granted. There are so many things that we appreciate more today because of the pain we experienced. Maybe it's just the realization of how special life really is. A lot of people don't even think about that because it's supposed to happen, meaning you're supposed to get married and have kids and have a family. We take things for granted along the way. Lisa and I don't look at things the same way anymore, things about us or about our children. Maybe that's the reason "why" it happened.

Plus, it's just nature. We're not the only ones this happens to, and it happens a lot. When things come together correctly and a healthy baby is born, it's unbelievable. But it's amazing that everything comes together right. There are so many things that could go wrong along the way. I never thought about that with my first child. I expected that he'd be healthy. Now, I think you're lucky when you can have a child.

About a year after we lost Daniel, Lisa and I were fortunate enough to have another baby together. Her pregnancy and delivery went smoothly. There were no complications like before. When he was born he was absolutely perfect. His name is Timothy. We're so thrilled to have a baby together. We really feel lucky that things finally worked out for our family.

~ **Michael**

Treatments for a Stillbirth

It's emotionally intense when you have to face the death of your fetus, regardless of its developmental stage. Once a stillbirth has been diagnosed there are options every couple must consider. A woman can choose to wait for her body to naturally go into labor. Without medication, it could take up to two weeks before her body gives birth. The other choice is to take medication to induce labor. Many couples choose to induce labor so they can begin the healing process. If a woman's cervix doesn't dilate enough for the pregnancy to pass, doctors often use a hormone called oxytocin to make the uterus contract and prepare the cervix for labor.[3]

Causes of Stillbirth

"I wonder what I did wrong." "Did I overexert myself and work too many long hours?" "Could it be that I didn't take enough prenatal vitamins?" "What could I have done differently?"

All parents want to know why it happened. Typically after a stillbirth delivery, the fetus, placenta, and umbilical cord are evaluated to determine cause of death. Many couples ask their doctors to do chromosomal analysis to find out if certain genetic disorders or infections caused the fetus's death. In some cases, autopsies are performed. Unfortunately, in almost 50 percent of cases the cause of death remains a mystery.

The most common causes of stillbirths include:
• problems with the placenta
• lack of oxygen
• insufficient nutrition
• genetic problems
• trauma
• high blood pressure
• infections
• problems with the umbilical cord

Smokers, alcohol and drug abusers, and women over the age of 35 are all at an increased risk for having a stillbirth. Women without prenatal care and those who don't eat healthy, balanced meals are also at a disadvantage when it comes to carrying a fetus to full term.

The good news is that the number of stillbirths has decreased in the United States over the past twenty years. Today women have access to better healthcare options, giving them the knowledge and resources to more likely maintain a healthy pregnancy and successful delivery. [3, 4]

CHAPTER THREE

what are you willing to do to have a baby?

Lesley and I had already experienced one failed pregnancy. The first one was a sneaky ectopic that showed few symptoms but ended up threatening her life. As a result, I felt guarded and almost pessimistic during our second pregnancy. I was worried Lesley might have a second tubal pregnancy.

~ Brian

My Second Pregnancy

After my first ectopic pregnancy, Brian and I waited four months before we tried again. It took us about seven months to finally conceive, but when I got pregnant the second time, I was very optimistic. I'd beaten the odds by getting pregnant via one good fallopian tube, so I thought, *Why wouldn't my pregnancy continue successfully?*

I was confident that my pregnancy would not turn into another ectopic. I assured Brian that things would be different. He tried to pretend he wasn't worried. I kept telling him that he was going to jinx my pregnancy if he wasn't excited about our new baby. I even convinced him to talk to my belly to encourage our fetus to fight for his life and make us proud parents. My hormone levels were low in the early weeks, a sure sign that something was wrong.

Nevertheless, I'd made up my mind to focus on the positive and believe everything was going to work out.

During week seven of my pregnancy, Dr. King broke the bad news that I was indeed having another tubal pregnancy. The only good news was that she caught it before my fallopian tube burst. She instructed me to go to the emergency room as soon as possible to have an injection of methotrexate, a drug to stop the growth of the pregnancy.[4] Dr. King said my fallopian tube wouldn't be damaged this time, since we'd caught it earlier than during my first pregnancy.

Again, my hopes were shattered. Now, with two pregnancy losses, I felt as though I had no control over my body. I realized that just because I wanted and dreamed about having a baby didn't mean it would manifest itself.

No amount of meditating or praying seemed to make a difference either. At times I felt peace, but I didn't sense that God was going to give me a baby. No angel appeared to me saying, "God has heard your prayers, Lesley. In due time you shall bear a child and the child shall be named John," or James or Sally Suzy for that matter. Nothing changed regardless of the Bible verses I claimed, asking God to bless me with a child just as He had blessed Sarah and Abraham in the Book of Genesis.

I was at a crossroads in my life and I needed to make a decision. My body had failed me twice. Should I give up the dream or listen to friends' advice and turn to modern technology?

Honestly, I was uncomfortable with the idea of using IVF. I was nine years old when Louise Joy Brown, the world's first successful "test tube" baby, was born in Great Britain. During my 20s I remember thinking that people who went to the extreme of having a test tube baby must be crazy. I never dreamed I would be faced with the decision to use the same technology myself.

Out of desperation, I decided to call Dr. Laura, the mother of wisdom and keeper of sage advice. I knew Dr. Laura would have no emotional involvement in my situation. I hoped she could give me a little perspective, at the very least. When I called Dr. Laura, the screener put me straight through to her. I was very nervous and didn't know exactly what to say or how to begin to explain my story. The following is the transcript from my phone conversation with Dr. Laura.

Looking for Answers

"1-800-D-r-L-a-u-r-a. Lesley, welcome to the program."

"Hi, Dr. Laura, thanks for taking my call."

"Thank you!"

"My question today is: I've had two ectopic pregnancies. With the first one I had laparoscopic surgery, and my second ectopic ended with an injection of methotrexate to dissolve the pregnancy. Now, my husband and I have gone to a fertility specialist looking into options. IVF, In Vitro Fertilization, would give us a 40 to 60 percent chance; 40 percent chance that it would work, 60 percent chance that it wouldn't work. So, I'm just having a really difficult time deciding if I would want to do IVF."

"Do you have a lot of extra money to spend on this? It's pretty expensive."

"Well, not a lot of extra, but we do have some money we could take out of savings. It would be fifteen grand, so that's a lot."

"But that's each time."

"Right, so we were thinking maybe we'd just do it one time and, if it doesn't work, then just be happy with what we have and be content and move on and quit dealing with this whole issue because it's been going on for three years of, *'Are we going to have a kid? Are we not going to have a kid?'*"

"So, do you still have your tubes?"

"I have one good tube and we also have sperm issues. But I have healthy eggs and a healthy uterus and ovaries. But he's got a low sperm count and motility issues. And I've got one tube. So, the doctor says we've got a 2 percent chance on our own each month to get pregnant. We keep trying and of course every month we're disappointed because it doesn't happen. After going through the emotional trauma of two ectopic pregnancies, I don't know if I can emotionally make it through the 60 percent chance of IVF not working out. And I just don't know whether or not to try it."

"How old are you?"

"Thirty-eight."

"You're almost 39 or you just turned 38?"

"I'll be 39 in February."

"Okay, we're closing in on a deadline here. You should sign up for an adoption and not put yourself through this."

"My husband is not into adoption."

"Perhaps you could go on the Internet or ask the doctor for some adoptive agencies and you can go to a group and meet people and he can talk about his concerns. He can hear back the experiences people have had. I'm just pointing out that there is another alternative because you're getting up in age."

"We know that's an alternative, but we figure that if we can't have one on our own..."

"Lesley, then flip a coin."

"Flip a coin?"

"Yeah. If it doesn't really matter and you have to take money out of savings and you know it's a low probability, then flip a coin."

"Cause you either take the risk or you don't?"

"Right."

"But it's just.... I don't know."

"Stop saying, 'I don't know.' There is no guarantee. There is only a shot in the dark."

"So, how do you know that you're going to get through that shot in the dark if it doesn't work? Emotionally?"

"Of course you're going to get through it. You've gotten through plenty of stuff in your life. You're not going to dissolve, like the Wicked Witch of the West. You're not gonna become a puddle."

"I like the analogy (laughing)."

"Yeah."

"Well, it's just so scary."

"Lesley stop saying, 'It's just so....' That's such an annoying phrase. Think about it. (mockingly, she says) 'It's just that I don't want…. It's just that I don't….' You're either going to jump in and take the risk or you're not. So flip a coin. But stop agonizing about it. You're not going to get any further agonizing about it. You're not going to get any further asking fifteen people their impression, because everybody has a different opinion of what they would like to go through. You're either going to try it or not. You're not gonna die from a loss."

"I just don't want to be a basket case if I don't…"

"You'll be a basket case for a little while and then you'll get over it. It's not terminal basket case-hood."

"Umm. It's just such a…"

"Stop, I don't want to hear anything you say after 'It's just.' That's so annoying."

"I'm sorry. It's a, it's a difficult decision. Let's put it that way."

"Flip a coin. Do you have a coin on you right now?"

"Um-mm. I can find one."

"Okay, I'll wait. Go ahead."

"There's one in the drawer, I'm sure."

"Good, I'll wait. Go get it."

"You can probably hear the drawer. There's a quarter."

"Good, that's heavy. Okay, heads is you're going to do it one time because you're not going to dissolve all your savings. You're going to do it one time. Tails is you're not and you're just gonna get a dog or a parakeet."

"We have a dog."

"A parakeet."

"Those are messy (laughing). Okay, I'm flipping it and it fell on the floor. What was it you said? Heads is what?"

"No, it has to come in your hand. So, you need both hands free. Heads is you're going to do it one time. Tails is you're not going to do it at all. So, I need you to put the phone in the crook of your shoulder."

"Got it."

"So, you need both hands. I need you to flip it. Catch it without looking. Put it on top of the other hand and tell me what it is."

"All right. Here we go. Oopsie. Well, it flipped when I did that; does that matter? All right. Let me do it again. Here we go. Oops. Now I dropped it on the floor. Okay. I'm not very coordinated."

"Well, obviously, yeah."

"It's... it's heads."

"Okay, so I guess you're gonna try it one time."

"Can I do it again?"

"No, you don't do it again until you get the answer you want. That's the answer. So you're gonna try one time."

"But I don't know if, I mean, I don't know if I want to do it again. I don't know if I want to do it."

"Okay, well you have a nice day now. I can't help you."

"So, you just think flip a coin and..."

"Yeah."

"Just go for whichever and don't worry about how you feel?"

"Right."

"Or worry about what happens?"

"Right."

"Don't worry about the 'what ifs?' Just do whatever?"

"So nobody should go into the Olympics because if they don't get the gold medal they're gonna feel bad so nobody should try anything?"

"No."

"Your mentality makes being human useless."

"It's just such a pain..."

"Stop saying, 'It's just.' I'm hanging up on you now. Bye. I'm Dr. Laura Schlessinger. Be right back. 'It's just...'"

Hard Decisions

Dr. Laura had a point. I needed to make a decision, but the thing that bothered me about the conversation is that she seemed so flippant about how I should make my decision. Surely I couldn't just flip a coin. The process and the outcome mattered too much. Maybe from her perspective it didn't matter. After all, who in their right mind calls a complete stranger asking her to solve their problems?

My call to Dr. Laura was an indication that I was seriously grasping for straws, looking for answers everywhere except the one place that mattered most. My heart. By talking to Dr. Laura, I realized that no one could make the decision for me. Going through the exercise of flipping a coin forced me to face my deepest fears. When the coin landed on heads, I realized that I wasn't ready to do IVF. I instinctively wanted to flip the coin again. I wanted the coin to land on tails. It was definitely a reality check. Even though I was uncomfortable with Dr. Laura's seemingly simplistic solution to my problem—"just flip a coin"—maybe she knew it would help me be honest with myself and stop me from trying to please everyone else. In that moment, I knew it was all about me, my body, and what I wanted to do. No one could make the decision for me.

Take Time

There have been times when I've felt lonely struggling through failed pregnancies, invasive surgeries, and numerous doctor appointments. Brian has stood by my side along the way, but he's not the one who has to crawl up on the exam table and be poked and prodded like a cow. He can only stand by and watch.

When you really don't know what to do, give yourself time to think. Time to process. Time to heal. Take baby steps. Even when doctors tell you that your biological clock is ticking, take a step back and breathe deeply. When I was torn apart by mental anguish and mixed emotions, I offered myself the gift of time. That was the best thing I could have given myself.

Seeking Wise Counsel

I was at my wits' end after two tubal pregnancies, so I found a counselor who specialized in women's fertility issues. I chose one with personal experience, as I figured that alone would be helpful to me. After telling her my story in a nutshell, she simply asked one question, "What do you want to do?"

I stared at her speechless, because I was completely out of

touch with my own feelings. I felt overwhelmed with everyone else's opinion, especially my husband's, who wanted me to do IVF. I didn't want to disappoint him or let him down. He really wanted a baby, as did I, but I was emotionally toast and my body had been through a lot already. I didn't know if I could endure countless hormone injections, weekly blood tests, and the many medical procedures that went along with the program.

I remember Brian pleading with me to do IVF.

"Just do it once, Lesley. I promise that if you do one cycle of IVF, then I'll never ask you to do it again."

Looking him sternly in the eyes I ranted, "IVF is unnatural. If I was supposed to have a baby, then it would have happened by now. I've already lost two children. But we just don't have anything to show for it—except for a lot of pain. Emotional and physical pain. Why do you want to play God and use artificial means to make a baby? You don't even know if IVF will give us a baby. The doctor said we only have a 40 percent chance at best if I did IVF. That's not very encouraging to me. Plus, I know you. You tell me now that if I did one cycle that you'd never ask me again. But if it didn't work out the first time I bet you'd ask me to do it again. So, when would it ever stop? How many times would you keep begging me to do IVF? How much do you want to put my body through just to have a kid? Where will you ever draw the line? Do you even know?"

"I don't know."

"Yeah, I didn't think so. You're not the one who has to endure needles being stuck in your butt on a daily basis, doctors poking around inside your vagina, having blood draws twice a week, and feeling terrible most of the time. Even after all that, who knows if we would even end up with a baby. The doctors can't make any promises."

"Well, a 40 percent chance with IVF is better than a 2 percent chance that we have on our own each month. Honey, I would be willing to do the injections for you, so you don't have to do that by yourself."

"Well, I guess that's more than most husbands are willing to do.

You know I love you, but I can't keep talking about this right now. Let's put it on the back burner for a while. Okay?"

"Okay, honey. We don't have to decide anything now. I love you and everything is going to be all right."

"I love you, too."

Sifting through My Feelings

I spent the next four weeks in counseling trying to sort out my thoughts and feelings. I sifted through my childhood dreams and adult visions for a family of my own. I talked about other goals of things I wanted to pursue, if I didn't have children.

In the midst of the confusion and pain, I realized that two pregnancy losses were not the end-all, be-all of my life. I could choose to focus on the positive or wallow in negativity and depression. Regardless of the path I chose, life would go on. The difference would be my attitude and how I approached life. Would I fight with clenched fists every situation I experienced? Or would I move on and embrace with open arms whatever life brought my way? The choice was mine and mine alone. No one could walk my journey for me. Dr. Laura knew that.

Finally, I was able to verbalize my true feelings. I told my counselor that I did not want to do IVF. It was a great relief just to say the words. She congratulated me on being honest with myself despite the outside pressures I felt. When I got home that day I told my husband.

"Brian, you know I've been thinking about this for months. It's been a heartrending decision but, at this time, I don't want to do IVF. There's nothing in me that wants to try it. The numbers aren't convincing for me but, regardless of that, I do not want to do it."

"Well, I'm not going to force you to do it. It's your body, and you would be the one who has to endure the physical part of doing IVF and then the pregnancy."

"I'm not saying I'll never do it. But for now, I don't want to do it. I hope you understand."

"I know it's been a tough decision for you. Honey, I love you and ultimately that is what matters. Us. You and me."

Working Towards a Resolution

It would be a perfect world if Brian and I agreed on everything. Who gets the bigger closet? Whose career is more important? Where to spend New Year's Eve? Things always come up—big and small—where we don't see eye to eye. How to approach our infertility issues is definitely a sensitive topic, and we haven't always agreed on decisions and solutions. Nevertheless, we have managed to keep our relationship primary and let everything else be secondary.

Early on in our marriage, we used silly tactics, like fussing, pouting, calling each other names, and using the silent treatment, to try and bend each other's will. That took too much energy. We finally learned to resolve our conflicts in a more mature manner. We wanted to do more than just get along. We wanted to thrive in our marriage. We yearned for an exciting relationship that would not grow dull through the years.

It was crucial for us to learn how to honor, respect, and trust one another on a deep, heart-felt level. It took intense emotional and mental work to make it happen, but we did it. Our secret to having an extraordinary relationship? Commit to find a Mutually Agreeable Decision (MAD). Instead of getting mad, use MAD.

We knew that, no matter how hard we tried to make mutually agreeable decisions, there would be disagreements because of opposing views, desires, or needs. Nevertheless, we learned how to find win-win solutions with one understanding: Each one of us must make sacrifices and be willing to concede selflessly. One thing is for sure: You can't always get what you want, but you can get close to what you need.

Don't Get Mad, Use MAD

The ground rules for finding a Mutually Agreeable Decision (MAD) are pretty simple. Commit to engage in four or five conversations and do a little soul-searching on paper. Answer the following "conflict resolution" questions:

- What do you think the conflict is?
- What do you believe your significant other thinks the conflict is?
- What can you do to resolve the conflict?
- What can your significant other do to resolve the conflict?
- What can you do to be more gracious and loving in this situation?

After we individually write down our answers to the questions, we share the results with each other. We listen with open minds, seeking to find a resolution to benefit both of us.

We've found this activity helpful because it keeps us from attacking one another. It gives us the opportunity to think through our thoughts before blurting them out in anger.

When we can't find an obvious solution, we push ourselves to think outside the box. We brainstorm on a separate sheet of paper, writing down additional ideas and listing alternative options. By no means are we perfect, but we're always amazed by the fresh ideas we create when working together in love, rather than against each other in anger.

Elizabeth's Story: How Far Will You Go to Have a Baby?

There are enormous emotional, physical, mental, and financial ramifications to consider when trying to start a family. There comes a point when you have to ask yourself: How far will I go to have a baby? What are we willing to sacrifice to have a child? It's a very personal and difficult decision. Elizabeth explains her experience.

Trying to have a baby affects you on every level— socially, emotionally, physically, and financially. My entire circle of friends and I were all trying to get pregnant. It turned into this unofficial competition of who could get pregnant first. One of the girls got pregnant and the next girl got pregnant—and then I had an ectopic pregnancy. Then the next girl announced a few days later that she was pregnant, and her husband said to me, "Ha, ha, we beat you!"

When another friend gave birth, I went to see the baby in the hospital. I started crying and almost couldn't stop. My husband, Paul, started giving me a hard time, saying I was a bad friend and a crazy person. I realized that I did need some help. I wasn't doing well. Going to ten baby showers wasn't making me feel any better either. Friends were always asking, "What's wrong with you and Paul; how come you're not having children?"

I went to see a therapist for five years straight during our infertility problems. We had a lot of marriage problems through all of it. It was so hard on our marriage. I was feeling so overwhelmed working full time, taking care of the house, and trying to have a baby.

I've been on a roller coaster of depression and grief. I gained a lot of weight. At one time I was over 200 pounds. One summer I spent thousands of dollars shopping. I was really depressed the whole time. Even though I was in therapy, I knew how to hide everything by buying things or eating whatever I wanted or working way too hard or deciding that I didn't want to work that much at all. It was a really weird time.

To pay for all of our assisted reproductive technology (ART) procedures, we refinanced our house and I exercised stock options I had with my employer. I made a lot of money on my stock options. We had savings, but we used all of that, so we started dipping into equity. We used everything that we felt comfortable with. We still have equity left in our house. We didn't go completely crazy with that, but our savings are depleted. We spent way too much. I have no more stock. My portfolio is gone. Even if Paul said let's try one more time, there is no more money to do it. I would have to apply for credit cards. There are ways to finance medical procedures like IVF or plastic surgery, but we didn't want to do that. We've been trying to rebuild."

~ Elizabeth

How to Choose a Fertility Specialist

Choosing a fertility specialist is a major decision. Not only is it expensive to use ART, it's also invasive. You need to be comfortable with the doctors and nurses with whom you will be interfacing on a weekly basis.

First, talk to your family doctor and OB-GYN and ask for a referral. Ask your friends for referrals and meet the doctors in person. Your first meeting with a fertility specialist will normally last about an hour. You can expect to fill out forms asking about your medical history. It helps to have a copy of your records with you. Take your insurance card and be prepared to discuss how you plan to pay for your services. Some doctors will even want to do a physical exam on your first visit. Just be prepared.

One of my friends, who had twin boys through a successful IVF cycle, suggested that I meet with her doctor. So, I made an appointment and was pleasantly surprised when I met Dr. Michael Kettel at the San Diego Fertility Center. During our first meeting with Dr. Kettel, Brian and I sat in his office talking for an hour. He was very professional, obviously brilliant, and very likable, and he answered all of our questions. Dr. Kettel didn't pressure us at all. I knew that if I ever decided to do IVF, Dr. Kettel would be my first choice for a fertility specialist.

Choosing to Use Fertility Treatments

It took me time to digest the pain of my first two ectopic pregnancies. I was also disillusioned when I learned through the HSG test that I had only one good fallopian tube. I was shocked and often thought, How could this be happening to me?

Although I told Brian that I didn't want to do IVF, I kept wondering about the possibilities. Would IVF work for me? Is a 40 percent chance of having a baby worth the risk? I don't respond well to being pressured; it clouds my thinking. My instinct is to say "no" just to be left alone. But since Brian wasn't expecting me to do IVF, I felt no pressure from him and, for the first time, I really felt free to seriously consider it as an option.

I knew the odds were slim. Dr. King had told us we had a 2 percent chance of conceiving each month on our own. Dr. Kettel said we had a 20 percent chance each year of getting pregnant without medical help. That fact alone made me stop and think twice.

I also knew my biological clock was ticking. The older I got, the older my eggs would be. I knew that if I was ever going to do IVF, now would be the best time.

Shopping helps me think. So, I took my credit card and went to the nearest mall.

I was in the dressing room at Anthropology, trying on a cobalt blue dress, when I made a definitive decision to try one IVF cycle. Standing in the dressing room, I dialed the fertility center on my cell phone and asked Dr. Kettel's nurse to sign me up and send a prescription to my pharmacy for birth control pills. I had read all the information and knew that, in order to begin IVF, I needed to start taking birth control pills on day 4 of my cycle. The nurse was excited for me and told me the prescription would be ready later that day. I had put the wheels in motion.

There were, however, still decisions to be made. Brian and I had not talked about what we would do with extra embryos if we had any. I figured that conversation could wait until I made my Anthropology purchase and saw him face to face. Little did

Brian know that I had made a big decision that also affected him. I knew he would love my blue dress, but I also knew he would be even more thrilled that I'd changed my mind about doing IVF. I grabbed my package and hurried home as fast as I could.

Before Meeting with a Fertility Specialist

I am a list-keeper. I write lists for house chores, books I want to read, movies I want to see, and menus I plan to cook. It's ridiculous how many lists I have taped to doors and mirrors. While facing fertility issues, it was only natural that I make a list of questions to ask the doctor. The list continued to grow, getting more complicated as we investigated our options.

When I first began considering fertility options, I was extremely concerned with the risks associated with the use of procedures such as intrauterine insemination (IUI), intracytoplasmic sperm injection (ICSI), and IVF.

I have noticed that couples who conceive easily rarely think about the risks associated with pregnancy. The fact is that there are always risks, such as birth defects, chromosomal abnormalities, and pregnancy complications for the mother. Birth defects occur in about 2 to 4 percent of all live births. They happen randomly, and there's no way to prevent them, though research shows that taking folic acid every day can help prevent spinal cord defects.

The causes of about 70 percent of birth defects are unknown. A single gene change can cause birth defects. Genes are contained in each of the 46 chromosomes inside our cells. Genetic abnormalities (such as hemophilia, cystic fibrosis, muscular dystrophy, color blindness, and Huntington's chorea) result when DNA mutations are passed on from a parent.

About 1 in 150 babies in the United States is born with a chromosomal abnormality. Chromosomal abnormalities usually result from an error that occurs when an egg or sperm cell develops. Egg and sperm cells each contain 23 chromosomes. When they join together, they form a fertilized egg with 46 chromosomes. But sometimes something goes wrong before fertilization. An egg or sperm cell may divide incorrectly, resulting in an egg or sperm cell with too many or too few chromosomes. Sometimes the embryo dies even before implanting in the uterus. Other times, the embryo will implant and die (possibly miscarry). More than 50 percent of first-trimester miscarriages are caused by chromosomal abnormalities in the embryo.

It is important to do your own research before meeting with a fertility specialist. It will save you time and money. You can find a lot of information at your local library, as well as online at web sites such as www.marchofdimes.com (March of Dimes), www.resolve.org (National Infertility Association), www.asrm.org (American Society for Reproductive Medicine) and www.theafa. org (American Fertility Association).

Questions You Can Find Answers to on Your Own
- How long has the fertility specialist been performing ART procedures?

- What is the fertility specialist's success rate with IUI, IVF, live births, etc.?

- What does the clinic charge for the services they offer, including treatments, drugs, follow-up visits, long-term freezing of embryos, and selective reduction? Call the clinic's financial/billing office to obtain specific information.

- What percentage of IUIs/IVFs end in ectopics? Miscarriages? Stillbirths?

- If the first ART cycle fails, what is the waiting period before doing another cycle?

- What is transvaginal egg retrieval?

- What is intracytoplasmic sperm injection?

- How does poor sperm quality affect the health of an embryo?

- When is testicular sperm retrieval recommended?

- Is it possible to increase sperm quality?

- How does age (quality of the eggs) affect the possibility of a pregnancy ending in a miscarriage or stillbirth?

- What is the shelf life of frozen embryos?

- Does the use of IUI or IVF increase the baby's risk for birth defects?

- After an embryo transfer, how long should I stay on bed rest?

- Are there restrictions on physical activity, hair coloring, travel, caffeine, alcohol, foods, medications, or herbal supplements?

Sixteen Important Questions You Might Want to Ask Your Fertility Specialist

Brian and I took time to contemplate our fertility options. We read about the available treatments and procedures. After learning as much as we could on our own, we prepared the following list of questions to ask our fertility specialist. This list is not intended to be exhaustive but offers a starting point. Not all of these questions may apply to you, but here are sixteen important questions you might want to ask your fertility specialist when considering ART:

1. What tests do you require before we begin our first ART cycle?

2. Based on our age, blood tests, sperm quality, and ultrasound results, what are our chances of having a live birth using ART?

3. What ART protocol do you recommend for our situation? Which drugs will you prescribe? Side effects?

4. Will you personally perform the ART procedures? If not, who will perform my blood tests, ultrasounds, egg retrieval, and embryo transfer? These are important questions because your doctor may be on vacation when it's time for your egg retrieval.

5. Do you offer sex selection? (Not all fertility clinics do.) If so, what procedure(s) do you use? What are the success rates? What are the risks?

6. If my first ART attempt is unsuccessful, will you continue working with me?

7. What is your protocol for testing my hormone levels during my ART cycle, to make sure my estrogen and progesterone levels are supporting the pregnancy?

8. Does genetic screening for various diseases negatively affect an embryo?

9. What are the side effects of the medications used to stimulate my ovaries? How do you keep from overstimulating my ovaries?

10. How do you determine the quality of my eggs?

11. How do you test for embryo viability? Negative effects?

12. Once my embryos develop, how much time will I be given to determine the number of embryos to transfer? Are there limits to the number of embryos you will transfer?

13. What options does your clinic offer regarding viable and non-viable embryos that are not transferred (e.g., freezing, destroying, donating)?

14. Does IVF increase my risk for ovarian cancer?

15. What are the chances and risks of having a multiple gestation pregnancy (e.g., triplets, quadruplets, or

more)?

16. Do you offer selective reduction (also called "multifetal reduction," used to reduce the number of embryos in the uterus) in house? What is your policy? Cost?

Jumping in with Both Feet: In Vitro Fertilization (IVF)

Since I decided to give IVF a shot (pun intended), I put all my fears aside and pushed forward hoping for the best. But as I sat in Dr. Kettel's office, my head began to spin, listening to long words like hysterosalpingogram, ovarian hyperstimulation syndrome, intracytoplasmic sperm injection, and blastocyst transfer. I needed a PhD just to understand what he was talking about.

When considering ART, find a really good dictionary or a friend in the medical field to help you decipher the medical terminology, or just sit back with a decaf latte and continue reading this chapter. The following section tells you what to expect regarding infertility treatments and procedures for women. Chapter 5 covers male infertility procedures. Several couples share their experiences throughout the following sections, offering easy-to-understand explanations of common ART procedures.

Rachel and Steve's Story: Intrauterine Insemination (IUI)

After getting married, Rachel and Steve expected their life would progress in the "normal" stages. First, they bought a house to remodel. Then they traveled the world and, in between destinations, talked about the two or three kids they wanted to have one day. Planning for the future, they even saved some money along the way. Rachel and Steve were in their mid-20s when they decided to start their family. Rachel shares their story.

When I was 18, I got pregnant with someone I was very much in love with, and he talked about marrying me because of the baby. He was a drug addict, and I knew there was no way things would work out, so I went into survival mode and had an abortion.

Two years later, I started developing an infection that turned into a mass in my abdomen. I was only 20 years old at the time. The mass was inside my fallopian tube, and it ballooned to the size of a cantaloupe. My other tube was infected and swollen to about the size of a lime. After removing the bad tube, they treated the infected tube. I was left with one tube, but my ovaries and uterus were unaffected.

Later, I met the love of my life and married him when I was 24. A couple of years late, Steve and I got pregnant. One day at work my breasts and nipples started to ache. I knew my body was withdrawing from the pregnancy. Blood came out in the toilet. I could barely stand up, but I had to push myself to get through the day; I couldn't leave work because I was the only manager that day. I was very upset about miscarrying my pregnancy.

Because of my medical history and the miscarriage, Steve and I found a high-risk pregnancy doctor who encouraged us to try IUI (a procedure in which sperm are "washed" to separate them from the semen and inserted, via a small tube, into the uterus after the ovaries have released one or more eggs).

The doctor said IUI would help separate the normal sperm from lower-quality sperm and increase the chances of Steve's sperm actually getting into my fallopian tube to fertilize an egg.

The doctor had already tested Steve's sperm to check its count, motility, and shape. His sperm were okay but they weren't great. Steve switched from briefs to boxers and quit taking hot showers to try and help his sperm quality improve. He was also under a lot of stress from his job at the time, so we knew that could hurt his sperm quality. We were willing to try anything the doctor said to do to have babies.

The doctor said that during intercourse only about 200 sperm out of 40 million actually make it past the cervical mucus into the fallopian tubes, where fertilization takes place. So, with IUI we could actually place 10 to 20 million sperm into my uterus near my one good tube, giving us a better chance of getting pregnant.

My doctor timed the IUI procedure to take place as close to my ovulation date as possible. I started taking Clomid, a fertility drug that stimulates your ovaries and helps the ovaries spit out more than one egg in a given cycle.

Steve gave his sperm sample, which he had been saving up for about five days. They say your count can be too low if you've just had sex a day or so before giving the sample. The doctors washed Steve's sperm to get it concentrated and more egg-friendly. Sperm have a higher pH than the vagina. Washing the sperm lowers the pH, making them more compatible with vaginal pH.

When my ovaries were ready to release my eggs, the doctor injected Steve's sperm directly into my uterus, helping the sperm get closer to my eggs to give those babies a fighting chance. The procedure is a lot like having a pap smear. They inserted a speculum in my vagina and inserted a catheter through my cervix to shoot the sperm up into my uterus.

Then, at that point, we just waited. It wasn't a painful procedure and I didn't have cramping or anything. Unfortunately, I didn't get pregnant. Months later I did two more rounds of IUI but never achieved a pregnancy.

I've always wondered if IUI didn't work because of my previously infected tube. Infections can cause scar tissue, and that impairs the hair-like structures from moving the egg and sperm through the tube. If the hairs can't move the egg and sperm down into the uterus, then you're out of luck. Maybe my eggs never made it down my tube to meet up with Steve's sperm.

Since fertility treatments failed for Steve and me, we eventually decided to look into other options, such as adoption, to start our family.

~ **Rachel**

Going from One Treatment to the Next

Once you've tried one ART procedure, should you move on to the next or quit? It's a very personal decision and a difficult one to make. Some people decide that after one ART treatment they want to stop. For one reason or another, they're just done. Others plow ahead and try again. Everyone is different. Consider what you've learned from the first ART treatment cycle. Did your ovaries respond to the fertility drugs? How many of your follicles contained viable eggs? Did the sperm wash improve the sperm's ability to penetrate the eggs? How did you feel during the cycle? What were your hormone levels? Did you have side effects from the hormone pills/injections? Knowing answers to these types of questions will help you think strategically about next steps. Discuss your results with your doctor to determine what's best for you.

I've learned that every treatment cycle should be looked at as an independent trial. I remember Dr. Kettel talking about the odds. He said that three IVF cycles would increase my chances of having a live birth. In other words, I had a 40 percent chance for success each time I did it and stressed that, if my first cycle didn't work, I had an equally good chance of a second cycle producing a live birth. I understood what he meant but, in my mind, I didn't think of doing IVF as a numbers game. I was hesitant to do it even once because it was such an emotional commitment for me.

"Lesley, you should give your treatment protocol three to four cycles to work. I want you to understand that, according to all of our clinical studies, it's unlikely that conception will happen after only one attempt. There are no guarantees, but I just want you to know how things usually go," Dr. Kettel explained.

In Vitro Fertilization (IVF)

The treatment process for IVF is very detailed and takes place in several steps. Before we could even start our cycle, Brian and I had to undergo tests to verify the health of my ovaries and uterus, his sperm quality, and my fallopian tube patency (openness of the tubes). Our insurance didn't cover anything, so our expenses for IVF were out of pocket. When Brian wrote the $10,400 check to our fertility doctor, I kept thinking about that money and how it could be used to pay down our mortgage. We began our IVF cycle in December. We were lucky because another patient donated an additional $4,000 worth of fertility drugs to us, which was like receiving a wonderful present.

We were given a lot of information to read. According to the experts, a woman's fertility starts to decline after the age of 35. She also has a higher chance for a miscarriage and chromosomal abnormalities. The Day 3 follicle-stimulating hormone (FSH) test offers more insight into reproductive health. FSH is a hormone that stimulates the ovaries to produce follicles, which contain one egg each. Not every follicle may contain an egg. It's a wait-and-see game. An FSH of less than 10 mIU/ml puts a woman in good standing for a successful IVF cycle. My test came back at 7.2 mIU/ml, which certainly gave me hope.

One point to note: A Day 3 FSH reading varies from one cycle to the next in every woman. I read a story in a fertility journal about a 43-year-old woman whose FSH was 12.4 mIU/ml. Nevertheless, she had a successful IVF cycle. So, FSH is not the only indicator of fertility health. Having a low FSH does not guarantee a successful pregnancy, but having a high FSH doesn't necessarily knock you out of the ball game either.

There are a lot of "rules" when doing IVF. No smoking. It decreases your fertility by 30 percent. Luckily that wasn't an issue for us. Only one cup of coffee per day. I could live with that. No alcohol because it decreases sperm count—something we certainly didn't want to risk. So we cut out wine, beer and liquor. When New Year's Eve rolled around we opted for sparkling cider. Brian could exercise but I wasn't allowed to play tennis. Dr. Kettel did, however, give me permission to walk and swim.

Since we needed to be organized to follow the rigorous daily schedule, we set up our hall bathroom as our command center for fertility treatments. We sanitized the faucets, drawer pulls, doorknobs, and countertops with alcohol, ensuring we killed every little germ. We lined the counter with bottles of alcohol, cotton balls, Q-tips®, scissors, Germ-X, Band-Aids®, sterile syringes, needles, gauze, and a needle disposal container. We were prepared.

On day 4 of my cycle, I began taking birth control pills to enable Dr. Kettel to coordinate my cycle with his treatment protocol. Every day, I religiously took a prenatal vitamin, an additional 4 mg of folic acid, and one baby aspirin, to increase my blood flow.

Then, the day arrived when Brian stepped up to the plate to deliver the first injection of Lupron, a hormone to prevent premature ovulation, into my abdomen. A nurse had taught him how. Initially I was terrified. The first time he inserted the needle into my stomach, it didn't hurt much. I only winced when he pulled the needle out at a 45-degree angle, leaving me bleeding and bruised. After a few more practice shots he perfected his technique. Brian continued giving me the shot every morning for 20 days.

After 23 days, I quit taking the birth control pills, per Dr. Kettel's orders. For the next three days Brian and I took Azithromycin (500 mg tri-pak) to eliminate bacteria that can be transmitted sexually. I had a short period for a couple of days, and then the nurse practitioner gave me a baseline ultrasound and blood tests to make sure my ovaries were not active.

Two days later Brian began giving me the first of eleven injections of Bravelle into my hip. By now he was an expert with needles. The injections weren't too bad unless he hit a nerve. Surprisingly, I only bruised a little from the shots. Bravelle is a hormone that stimulates the ovaries to make multiple follicles. Most people produce 10–15 eggs after being on Bravelle.

As my follicles grew larger and larger, I felt bloated, as if I had eaten too many cookies. But I was really glad that I didn't experience any of the other possible side effects, such as headaches, mood swings, or fatigue. Thankfully, other than the bloating, the hormones made me feel really good.

There are some less common side effects of taking Bravelle. Some women experience ovarian hyperstimulation syndrome, a condition in which the ovaries become swollen and painful. Depending on her condition, a woman's cycle may have to be canceled. Fewer than 2 percent of women taking fertility drugs develop a more severe form of ovarian hyperstimulation syndrome, which can cause rapid weight gain, abdominal pain, vomiting and shortness of breath. There's also a 25 percent chance that Bravelle will cause a woman to have multiples or even an ectopic pregnancy. The good news is that Bravelle doesn't increase the risk for birth defects.

A couple of days before my egg retrieval, I had an ultrasound. I asked the nurse to write down my follicle count and size. My right ovary had eight follicles growing. Two of the follicles were 19 mm, one follicle was 18 mm, another was 15 mm, and the other was 14 mm. My left ovary contained nine follicles: 24 mm, 20 mm, 15 mm, 12 mm, and 11 mm. The whole process amazed me.

Brian also gave me a one-time injection of Ovidrel, a hormone that induces ovulation when the follicles are mature, 36 hours before my egg retrieval.

On day 12 my follicles were ready to be harvested. Brian provided a semen sample within one hour of my scheduled egg retrieval. He shares his experience.

The instructions were clear: Abstain from sexual activity for at least three days, then produce the sample without lubes, saliva, or other bodily fluids.

"Dry rub," I joked with Lesley. "I'll bet doctors have all kinds of stories of what they've found in semen samples."

I was driving to the doctor's office before work with my sample in a brown paper bag, sitting in my lap to make extra sure it would arrive safely. I had at least 20 minutes to get it there before the sperm would, what, curl up and die? I wasn't sure, but I prayed I wouldn't hit much traffic. I did. About 15 minutes later I arrived. I ran into the hospital and down the stairs to drop off my semen sample, a mere five minutes to spare.

There were two receptionists, but both were busy with patients. 'Dammit!' I thought to myself. Tick, tick, tick. I checked my watch. Time was running out quickly. I was seriously thinking of butting in and depositing my semen when the other person stepped aside. I hurried to the receptionist's desk.

"I have a...ummm...sample to drop off," I said producing the bag, because I was ready to get out of there.

"What is it exactly?" the nurse asked.

"Semen. Semen sample," I replied as the elderly woman at the next window glanced over at me.

"And who is it for?"

"Dr. Kettel."

"Oh, he's not here. You'll need to go down that hall and turn left. Next patient?"

Damn! Time's almost out!

I ran down the hall to another receptionist's desk. Panting and no longer timid, I almost shouted as I held the bag up, "Semen sample for Dr. Kettel!"

She gave me a "get you and your semen out of my face" look and said, "Not here, go in through that door on your left."

I raced through the door and finally found someone who would take my semen. Whew! I'd just made it in time.

~ **Brian**

I was given anesthesia for the retrieval procedure. Dr. Kettel retrieved fourteen follicles from my ovaries, but only six follicles contained mature eggs. I was pretty disappointed after all the work and effort I'd contributed to the whole process. Typically, about 80 percent of the follicles from the ovaries will contain eggs.

The embryologist fertilized all six of my eggs with Brian's sperm, using a procedure called Intra Cytoplasmic Sperm Injection (ICSI). ICSI is used when the sperm have a difficult time penetrating the eggs. Using a needle, the embryologist places one sperm in each egg. Because I only had six eggs, they used ICSI to give us the best possible outcome. Regardless of whether you use natural fertilization or ICSI, fertilization occurs in about 60 percent of the eggs. Unfortunately, one of my eggs fertilized abnormally and three of the eggs didn't fertilize at all. Luckily, the other eggs fertilized perfectly, giving us two healthy embryos.

Three days after my egg retrieval, my embryos were ready to be transferred back into my uterus. The transfer took place in one of the regular exam rooms at our fertility clinic. The nurses turned out all the lights in the hallway and in my exam room, explaining that embryos don't like bright lights. I imagined my embryos crying out, "Bright light, bright light!" just like Gizmo from Gremlins. My embryos were brought into the room in a sealed container, and the doctor quickly inserted them into my uterus. From start to finish the procedure only took 10 minutes. We could see the injection taking place on the ultrasound monitor. I had to blink back my tears so I could watch the screen. I didn't want to miss anything. It was a miracle to see my itty-bitty embryos on the monitor. I knew they had to be tough little critters to have made it this far. I hoped they would grow quickly, so Brian and I could welcome them into our lives.

For the next three days I hung out in bed, playing cards, reading, and watching movies. I focused on positive thoughts, willing our embryos to implant and to grow inside my womb. I took a small pill called Prednisone, to keep my body from rejecting the embryos, and an antibiotic, Doxycycline, to prevent infection. Brian pulled out the big needles and starting giving me intramuscular injections of progesterone to support implantation of the embryos. It all seemed like a science project.

"That needle is big! That's gonna hurt," I said as Brian filled the needle with progesterone.

"Well, it's got to be done."

"Hey, I think you're actually enjoying this. Aren't you?"

"Well, I sure do love the view. Come on, turn around and bend over."

About sixteen days after my eggs were retrieved, I had my first pregnancy test. Brian and I prepared for the news, good or bad, by putting two bottles on ice: Rotari Riserva, my favorite champagne, and Martinelli Sparkling Cider. If the pregnancy test was negative we planned on getting drunk, but if it was positive we would toast our success with apple cider.

We were thrilled to hear that my pregnancy test was positive. Dr. Kettel said one of my embryos implanted and was growing successfully. For a moment we mourned over the embryo that died, wishing it could have lived. The weeks passed. During week four we saw our fetus's heartbeat. Finally, we were going to have a baby. It was exciting to see technology at work, helping us make our dreams come true.

I watched the ultrasound monitor. Here it was, the moment in "Peanuts" where Charlie Brown is sure he's going to kick the football this time, only to have it yanked out from under him in another defeat. But instead of an empty womb, I saw something incredible. It was our baby, peanut-shaped and tiny.

"There it is," the technician said, probably for the hundredth time, but pretending to be enthusiastic. "Do you two see the heartbeat?"

And I did see the heartbeat! A rhythmic flutter on the screen, "beat...beat...beat." My God, there was our baby and it was alive. I tried to hold back tears as I stared with amazement at the ultrasound.

I didn't want this to stop.
 "Do you want a printout?"
 "Yes!" I blurted out a bit too eagerly.
 There was our baby—finally. I gazed at the ultrasound printout all evening, hardly believing it.

~ Brian

After nine weeks, I graduated from the fertility clinic, saying good-bye to the nurses and Dr. Kettel. I also quit taking progesterone injections.

I found an OB-GYN named Dr. Gerber, thinking it was an appropriate name for my baby's doctor. I went to my first appointment to establish a relationship and to get Dr. Gerber up to speed on my pregnancy. Brian didn't go to the doctor's appointment because he was in an engineering management program and had class that day. We'd been feeling like a normal pregnant couple ever since we graduated from the fertility clinic.

Dr. Gerber asked how I was feeling and began doing the transvaginal ultrasound. As I lay on the exam table, I waited in anticipation, wondering how much longer my little fetus would be this week.

"Dr. Gerber, how does my baby look? I've already seen the fetal heartbeat three times at the fertility clinic. My last appointment was a week ago on Monday."

"Well, I am not seeing a heartbeat right now. Let me move the ultrasound device around to get a better angle."

Seconds passed.

"I still don't see a heartbeat. I don't see any movement. I'm sorry."

I was stunned speechless.

"Sometimes its difficult to get a clear picture. Let me call the fertility clinic and talk to them. I'll be right back."

I waited, feeling like I was frozen in time. I thought about Brian sitting in class and that I needed to call him. I wanted him to be with me.

Dr. Gerber came back into the room. "Lesley, I'm actually

going to send you over to another office just around the corner that has 3D ultrasound. It will give us three dimensional images of the fetus. I'm making an appointment for you this afternoon. You can get dressed now."

I pulled on my jeans and slipped my toes into my flip-flops. After getting into my car, I texted Brian, "Call me ASAP. Urgent."

A minute later my cell phone rang. "Lesley, where are you?"

"I'm sitting in the parking lot at the doctor's office," I said, as my voice trailed off and in a whisper I added, "You've got to come home."

"Are you okay?"

"No, Dr. Gerber said there was no heartbeat," I mumbled between sobs. "She couldn't find a heartbeat. Now, she's sending me to another office with a 3D ultrasound machine to see what's wrong. Our appointment is in a couple of hours."

"Can you drive home?"

"I don't know. I guess."

"Take it slow. Just drive home and wait for me. I'll be there as soon as I can. I love you."

"Okay."

I took the back roads home. Once I arrived I sat on the patio and waited for Brian. Time stood still. Nothing mattered anymore. I felt dead. I didn't want to breathe. I wanted my heart to stop. I didn't want to face the inevitable misery lying at my door, waiting for me to pick it up and embrace it. Cruel misery. I shuddered at the idea of coping with another loss. Devastation. Pain. Depression. I knew we were about to enter hell once again. Black. Dark. A dreadful place to be. A place where I want to lash out and curse God. A place where I have no control. Crazy thoughts passed through my mind as I began the gradual descent into depression's depths.

I spoke out loud, hoping God would answer. "How are we going to make it? How are we gonna get through this one? Again? We've seen the heartbeat three times. Is this really happening? Maybe the machine is just old. Maybe the doctor is wrong."

Silence surrounded me, except for the birds chirping in our pomegranate tree. The tree that Brian would harvest in November, the same month our baby was supposed to be born. I continued waiting.

From behind me I heard the patio door slide open. I stood and turned towards Brian, grabbing him as tight as I could. We held each other and sobbed.

"Our appointment is at 1 p.m., so we don't have a lot of time. We'd better go."

> We entered the building where Lesley would be scanned by the "high-tech" ultrasound. I noticed that there were several cancer center offices too. Brightly colored murals lined the walls, trying to offer hope for a better day. Damn, there must be a hell of a lot of misery in this place, I thought.
>
> I still held out faint hope that the other ultrasound had just missed something, that we'd hear, "Oops, our bad, everything is okay after all. You're baby's fine! Sorry for the scare."
>
> The lights were dim in the ultrasound exam room. A girl, probably in her mid twenties, was there to run the equipment. She started the process. I sat facing the computer monitor. Lesley laid on the table and couldn't see anything but a blank wall.
>
> The machine was bad-ass. No missed diagnosis with this thing. Not only did it show a clear image on the screen, it also had audio and scanned like radar for any movement that would give even a hint of a heartbeat. The fetus was there, but it was completely still. No flitter at all.
>
> "Do you see anything?" Lesley asked.
>
> There was nothing. I knew it and the girl knew it, but she followed strict protocol. "Dr. Gerber will go over all the details with you. I'm just the ultrasound technician."
>
> "But can you see a heartbeat?" Lesley pressed on.
>
> "No," she finally admitted.
>
> Our baby was gone. We left the doctor's office. I comforted Lesley but felt like I'd been smacked on the

head by a two-by-four and, mostly, just numbly stared
ahead.

~ Brian

Dr. Gerber said I experienced symptoms of a miscarriage. I was at 9½ weeks. A few days later she performed a D&C, saying they could test my pregnancy material to determine potential genetic abnormalities. Unfortunately, the test results didn't make us feel any better. They only showed that there was nothing genetically wrong with our fetus. We had no idea why our baby's heart had stopped.

I stayed home from work, not wanting to face the world. I was devastated. I ignored phone calls and emails, sleeping as much as possible to escape the mind-wrenching reality that slapped me in the face each time I opened my eyes.

A few days after my D&C, I woke up in the middle of the night to go to the bathroom. I didn't want to wake Brian, so I walked down the hall to the guest bathroom. Sitting on the commode I felt a knife-like pain in my abdomen. It literally took my breath away. I had never felt that kind of throbbing discomfort. As I tried to push myself up from the commode, I remember thinking I've got to get back in bed. Then, my mind went blank.

When I woke up, my mind was fuzzy. Vision blurred. I felt disoriented and confused. Paralyzed. I wanted to cry out for help. Silence surrounded me. My arms wouldn't move. My head throbbed. A fog surrounded me. My body trembled. I felt cold. My panties were twisted around my ankles. Then, I could feel something warm running down my inner thighs.

Finally, through the pain I mustered enough strength to moan, "Uuuuuuugg."

In the middle of the night, I heard a boom and it
woke me up. Feeling groggy, I raised my head from the
pillow. I wondered if someone was trying to break into
the house. I looked over at Lesley. She was gone. I
thought, It's just her bumping around in the bathroom.

90

I sunk down into my pillow, about to drift back off to sleep.

Then, I heard a muffled groan, "Uuuuuuugg." Something was definitely wrong. I got out of bed to look for Lesley. I rushed to the hall bathroom and found her lying on the floor on her right side.

Kneeling down and rolling her over towards me I asked, "Are you okay? What happened?"

She didn't respond.

"Oh, my God!" Leaning closer, I saw the entire right side of her face covered in blood.

"Lesley, what happened!?"

She only stared straight ahead with her mouth open. Then her whole body convulsed and shivered. I was really scared. I ran back to the bedroom and grabbed the phone and called 911 while I raced back to her. It was 4 a.m. and I got right through to the operator.

"My wife is on the floor and she's bleeding!"

"Sir, find a blanket and cover your wife. Do not move her. You understand?"

"Yes."

"I'm connecting you with the paramedics, now. Please hold."

The paramedics also told me to keep Lesley lying down and that they would be on their way. I found a blanket and covered her. I pulled up her underwear and adjusted her nightgown, getting her ready for strangers to carry her out. I got a wet cloth to clean her face. I was thankful to see that the bleeding was from a cut above her eye and seemed under control. She was somewhat conscious, and I instructed her to stay lying down.

Amazingly, the paramedics arrived in just over five minutes, an ambulance and fire truck with lights on but sirens silent. I led them upstairs. Our dog, Baby, barking behind the closed bedroom door, was finally awake and sensing that things weren't right in our house.

The paramedics examined Lesley. She had a head injury, so they brought in a stiff board to move her to the ambulance.

"Miss, can you tell me your name?"

"Lesley."

"Can you tell me where you are?"
"I don't know. Home I guess."
"Can you tell me what happened?"
"No."
As she finally regained consciousness, she asked,
"Do I have to go? I wanna stay home. I'm a tough
cookie."
"No, you could have head trauma and we need to
take you to the emergency room."
The paramedics taped her to the board and brought
her down the stairs. I noticed her hand keeping her
nightgown from riding up. Even in her semiconscious
state, she was still modest. I took it as a good sign,
but I was still scared and concerned. Did she have a
concussion? Would she be okay? So many questions
as I drove down the street, following the ambulance to
the hospital.
"God, let her be okay," I prayed.

~ Brian

I remember Brian hovering over me with a panicked look on his face that night. He was talking, but his words didn't register in my mind. I couldn't speak. My thoughts were jumbled, and for a while I had no sensation in my arms or legs.

My fall in the bathroom left me with on-going migraines and a major concussion that affected my memory. Details escaped me. If Brian asked me to buy milk at the store, I would forget to do it. I couldn't recall details about past events and conversations with friends. It took roughly a year to fully recover my memory.

Dr. Gerber said the excruciating pain that caused me to faint that night was probably triggered by a blood clot resulting from my D&C.

Brian and I were devastated by the miscarriage, but the bathroom incident made life even more difficult. We were so emotionally raw that we decided to take some time off from our baby-making endeavors. We decided to plan a fun trip somewhere, just to get away from all the drama.

CHAPTER FOUR

looking for answers: holistic techniques to help increase fertility

Holistic fertility treatments go beyond treating your reproductive organs to treating your whole being—mind, body, and soul. Your sense of mental well-being, level of physical fitness and connection to your emotional and spiritual bedrock impact your fertility health. Acupuncture, massage therapy, guided imagery, meditation, and prayer are all examples of holistic alternative treatments. Many couples have found these complementary therapies a welcome adjunct to their focus on increasing fertility.

The Wonders of Acupuncture

I don't necessarily like sharp objects, but there's something about having a hundred needles stuck in my skin that elevates me to a Zen-like state. Acupuncture helps me transcend the material world into tranquility. A state of bliss. No pain. No memory. No fear. No anger. Actually, very few thoughts or feelings whatsoever. Timeless space where I mentally float along in peace. Harmony fills every cell of my being. Clarity flows through my veins. Maybe it's the fact that I'm forced to lie still for sixty minutes. I am forced to pause my rushing thoughts and just be. Everything slows down, including my heartbeat, blood pressure, and body temperature.

There is one downside. I've learned that moving is not a good idea when needles are stuck in my torso, arms, and legs. During my first acupuncture appointment, my nose started itching and I instinctively raised my arm to scratch. Ouch! The needles in the bend of my arm dug deeper, hitting a nerve, which caused bleeding and an ugly purple bruise. Lesson learned.

Initially, I started going to an acupuncturist because I was seeking preventive treatment in between my migraine attacks. Acupuncture is thought to have positive affects on the balance of blood flow and Qi (also chi; means "life force" or "energy") throughout the body. During a migraine, blood vessels in the brain increase in size causing the headache. Acupuncture helps to regulate the flow of blood to the brain. It helped reduce the number of migraine attacks I experienced. Acupuncture is also thought to improve fertility.

What Is Acupuncture?

When I heard that acupuncture could improve men's and women's fertility by increasing blood flow to reproductive organs, I was intrigued. To learn more, I attended the Fertility Expo in San Diego. During one of the seminars, I met Marc Sklar, a Doctor of Acupuncture and founder of the Reproductive Wellness Clinic in San Diego. He explained everything I wanted to know about fertility acupuncture.

> *In acupuncture, to affect the health of the body, we use filaments, which are like needles, but they are actually solid all the way through. By inserting filaments into the body, we can regulate the nervous system and increase blood circulation. The general theory of acupuncture is based on the premise that*

there are patterns of energy flow (Qi) through the body, which are essential for health. Disruption of this flow is believed to be responsible for disease. Acupuncture can correct nervous system and blood flow imbalances at identifiable points close to the skin.

It takes about twelve weeks for the body to respond to fertility acupuncture treatment. One of the many reasons for the twelve-week mark is because the body requires a minimum of three months to make the necessary changes in female factor hormonal imbalances. Concurrently, the maturation and selection of eggs also takes sixty to ninety days.

This three-month minimum time period is especially important if a woman is also undergoing assisted reproductive technology, such as IVF. We have studies that show the benefit of optimizing a woman's endocrine system at least ninety days prior to any transfer procedures. It is during this time that her follicles are developing and, consequently, it is the best time to improve the quality of her follicles, verses only focusing on increasing the follicular quantity.

When it comes to male infertility, new sperm generation takes about the same ninety days. It will take this amount of time to begin affecting potential male factor abnormalities, such as low count, motility, or morphology issues.

For this, and many other reasons, the very minimum amount of time necessary to affect a meaningful change in a person's reproductive system is three complete menstrual cycles, or ninety days. If this is achieved, there will be an increased probability of conception. Acupuncture helps tremendously with low sperm count; we can make a big difference with poor motility or poor morphology, depending on the

disparity of it.
~ **Marc Sklar, LAC, DA, Founder of the**
Reproductive Wellness Clinic

Rebecca's and Erica's Stories: Acupuncture

A lot of women use acupuncture because it gives them a sense of control and the satisfaction of doing something positive for themselves. Those who use acupuncture before and after an embryo transfer during an IVF cycle have a 43 percent conception rate. Women not using acupuncture have a 26 percent rate, according to recent studies[5].

Research shows acupuncture's value in helping men and women who struggle with infertility. Rebecca, a 32-year-old graphic designer, shares her experience.

> *For a long time I have suffered from anxiety and depression because of my infertility problems. I have used Clomid for the past two years, trying to get pregnant without any success. Without Clomid I don't normally ovulate. A friend told me about acupuncture. After six months of using acupuncture along with herbal supplements, I finally got pregnant. It's a wonder treatment! Acupuncture has helped me relax and has had positive effects on my ability to conceive. I am now in my third trimester and feel great.*
>
> ~ **Rebecca**

Erica, a 27-year-old high school teacher, began using acupuncture before her third IVF cycle began. Never being able to achieve pregnancy before, she hoped a holistic approach of eating right, moderate exercise, and acupuncture would improve her chances for conception and a successful delivery.

My sister used acupuncture for her pregnancy and said she didn't get any nausea or vomiting while she was pregnant. That encouraged me to try it.

About eight weeks before my third IVF cycle was scheduled to begin, I started acupuncture treatments twice a week. My specialist said acupuncture would help increase blood flow to my uterus, tubes, and ovaries. It's also known to reduce the chance of miscarriage in the first trimester. I liked doing something beneficial for me in conjunction with my IVF cycle.

Acupuncture worked and I got pregnant. I used it throughout my pregnancy, and I feel like acupuncture helped move my body along towards the birthing process, when it was time to deliver my baby. Once my contractions started, things happened pretty quickly. Within seven hours of being at the hospital, I had given birth naturally without any drugs.

~ **Erica**

Rhonda's Story: Fertility Massage

I first heard about fertility massage at a support group where I met Massage Practitioner Genevieve Siegel of Gen-Touch Massage and Holistic Therapy and Reproductive Wellness. Many couples use it to improve their reproductive health, particularly the Maya Abdominal Massage. This massage removes or reduces blockages and impediments to the normal functioning of the female and male reproductive organs. The Maya Abdominal Massage is an external, non-surgical massage that helps treat, improve, and correct disorders in the digestive and reproductive organs. It helps women who have been diagnosed with forms of fallopian tube obstruction, abdominal adhesions, or endometriosis.

My acupuncturist told me about her patients

who had positive results using fertility massage to stimulate the reproductive organs, such as fallopian tubes and ovaries. I hoped it could help me, so I started getting them. It was like a regular massage, but the therapist used a smooth motion and not a lot of pressure. She massaged my stomach, applying pressure from my left hipbone up to my belly button, then repeated the same motion on the other side. I had it done right before I ovulated to increase my chances for having more follicles.

~ **Rhonda**

The female body experiences a lot of stress, as it goes through the changes experienced during pregnancy. Sometimes the changes can be uncomfortable. Fertility massage focuses on alleviating that stress in the body and can help improve flexibility and sleep, control blood pressure, release endorphins, and relieve muscle pain or fatigue.

Maya Abdominal Massage improves reproductive organ function and increases blood flow to the organs by releasing physical and emotional congestion or blockage in the abdomen. Congestion can be caused by previous surgeries that leave behind scar tissue. Endometriosis can cause blockage. If the uterus is affected by scar tissue or not in the right position, the reproductive organs will be out of balance. Sometimes the uterus will be out of position from women wearing high heels, running miles and miles, or having numerous childbirths. I focus on the front and back of the abdominal area, working to get the pelvis aligned, as well as getting congestion out of the abdominal and back area. Once we get the pelvis and other organs aligned, the uterus can get straightened out. When it is straightened out and in the proper position, the uterus can communicate with the ovaries, which communicate with the brain, to send the right amount of hormones.

It's estimated that 30 percent of woman who have been unsuccessful in conceiving, eventually conceive after a succession of Maya treatments. It's effective for both men and women.

~ Genevieve Siegel, HHP, LMT, Certified Practitioner of the Arvigo Technique of Maya Abdominal Therapy

Megan's Story: Guided Imagery

Guided imagery improves the mind-body connection. It allows the conscious mind to sync up with the subconscious, enabling the two to transfer information back and forth. Dr. Lorretta Shughrue, a San Diego-based counselor offering hypnotherapy programs to improve people's quality of life, explains how guided imagery works.

Guided imagery uses hypnosis to access the part of the mind, the subconscious, that is responsible for beliefs that motivate not only behaviors, but also emotional responses to situations. By using guided imagery, you can eliminate beliefs that are sabotaging your efforts and create new ones that allow you to positively transform your life. Using guided imagery relaxes the mind and helps you heal, learn, and create. It expands your ability to achieve your goals, putting you in control of your emotions and thought processes. My patients say it improves their attitudes and helps them form good habits.

~ Dr. Lorretta Shughrue

After five unsuccessful cycles of IUI, Megan learned that she had Polycystic Ovarian Syndrome (PCOS), a hormonal disorder that made her menstrual cycles irregular. A polyp in her uterus had to be surgically removed, leaving her with scar tissue. Her fertility specialist said she had a small chance of getting pregnant.

Desperately wanting to have a biological child, Megan and her husband decided to do another cycle of IUI using a holistic approach. That's when Megan began using fertility massage and guided imagery to help her achieve pregnancy.

To improve my chances of getting pregnant with IUI, I used guided imagery at the same time I did fertility massage. Guided imagery helped me focus my thoughts on accepting a new life and harboring a child. Before I went to sleep at night, I used guided imagery CDs to help me visualize the embryo and sperm coming together and swimming through my fallopian tubes. It taught me how to relax my thoughts and get focused on a baby coming into my life. I truly believe fertility massage and guided imagery helped me prepare for pregnancy. Both techniques were so relaxing, and they encouraged my body to work with my mind to make the pregnancy happen.

Before I started fertility massage and guided imagery, I felt like my reproductive system was stagnant. I believe the holistic approach helped open up my fallopian tubes, allowing my eggs to travel down and get fertilized. The massage got my blood flowing to my reproductive organs, making them function better.

When my nurse called to tell me I was pregnant, I was so excited. Now, I have a beautiful healthy baby to prove that IUI along with fertility massage and guided imagery works.

*~ **Megan***

What's Your Mental State?

Do you feel overwhelmed? Are you mentally fatigued? Is stress keeping you awake at night? How well are you functioning, day to day at work and in your relationships? Are you depressed? If you answered "yes" to any of these questions, stress may be taking a toll on you. Did you know that stress may cause your body to produce certain hormones that increase your risk for a miscarriage?

Feeling at peace and letting go of stressful thoughts in your life supports getting pregnant and maintaining a healthy pregnancy. Think about your lifestyle and daily obligations. If you work, how many hours are you clocking? What work or community activities are keeping you busy? Are you overcommitted in any of these areas? If so, where can you cut back to reduce stress in your life? Focus on finding a balance in your work, home, and social life, to allow yourself time to relax and unwind.

Being Present

What's your internal drama? Have you ever noticed the little voice in your head that is always talking? It chats incessantly about things that don't really matter. My little voice likes to focus on things in the past that have stressed me out. It replays stressful experiences repeatedly, telling me what I should have said or done. My little voice worries about things in the future. It creates scenarios that may or may not happen.

How does the little voice work? The little voice dumps junk thoughts into your stream of consciousness. Peace and joy get blocked out. When your mind is cluttered, there is no room for love to enter in and heal you. We need to discipline ourselves to practice a mindful presence.

Focusing on the present moment is the best way to stop the chattering little voice. I try to be aware of what is going on in my mind, refusing to allow negative thoughts to fill my consciousness. I've learned that the best way to stop the voice is to focus on my task at hand, such as working, walking my dog, or visiting with a friend. When focusing on the present moment, I give myself the gift of freedom and grace—freedom from past mistakes and grace for present living.

You'll find that it becomes easier to ignore the chatty little voice in your head as you touch, taste, see, hear, and smell the present moment. Realistically, the present moment is all you have. The past is gone. The future is not promised. We only have this moment. This present moment. Breathe in. Enjoy it. Make it count.

Meditation Helps You Focus on the Present Moment

Meditation is a very ancient and holistic practice that helps to reduce stress in life and work. It allows you to get beyond typical "thinking" and into a deeper state of mental relaxation. It can increase your ability to focus on the present moment. Meditation can reignite your spirit. The idea behind meditation is to sit silently and allow the imagination to quiet down. In the silence, you let go of all thought processes, allowing peace to dwell within.

How to Meditate

1. Sit comfortably in a quiet place away from distractions. Sometimes I sit on a yoga mat and other times I recline on my sofa under a blanket. Find a comfortable position, but don't be so relaxed that you fall asleep.

2. As you begin, state your intention to place yourself in a peaceful state of mind. Become aware of your breathing. Invite peace into your heart and seek clarity of mind. My one-sentence intention goes something like this: "In this moment, may I be open to peace and love as I quiet my thoughts and release all my cares. So be it."

3. Choose a special word to represent your intention of being present and at peace. It doesn't matter what word you choose. You can use a word like "love," "peace," "hope," or "joy," but you can also use words without any religious or spiritual meaning, including "rainbow," "flower," or "sky." Use a word that symbolizes your desire to enter a deeper state of awareness. Use your word to keep you focused when your imagination tries to take over. Each time

your mind wanders, just say your word quietly to yourself. You can expect outside thoughts to cross your mind. It's normal to be distracted. You might hear a car horn blowing on the street outside your window. You may even recall an annoying conversation you had with a friend. Just repeat your word and allow the thoughts to drift away as easily as they appeared. Try not to be upset by the thoughts. Just let them go effortlessly. Open your heart to peace and love during the silence and in the midst of your passing thoughts.

Depending on your ability to sit still, try spending fifteen to twenty minutes at a time in meditation. The fruit of your quiet time may not be evident at first, but give it time. Don't judge your experience based on how long you meditated or how many thoughts you ignored. The result of meditation will be seen in your attitudes and feelings. How peaceful do you feel? How loving are your actions and words? Do you have "Aha!" moments? Are you less stressed?

Prayer

About 90 percent of Americans pray everyday, according to recent studies. The beauty of prayer is that it can be done anytime and anywhere. Whether you are at the doctor's office, driving down the road in your car, or at work, God is only a breath away. Praying to God, or to your Infinite or Higher Power, offers many benefits when you're struggling with infertility. Most people feel an inner peace after prayer as it removes anxiety. Prayer can also be used as a catalyst for change in oneself. It can shift your perspective into a more positive attitude. Other benefits of prayer include:

- Better thought control and less intrusive thoughts
- Fights depression
- Increases overall sense of well-being
- Increases mental clarity and positive thinking
- Helps promote a restful night's sleep

Integrating holistic therapies, such as acupuncture, fertility massage, guided imagery, meditation, and prayer, may help increase your ability to conceive and carry a baby to full term. Holistic therapies give many men and women a positive way to proactively improve the health of their bodies and minds. It is to be hoped that these methods will help your mind and body get ready for pregnancy. It's a personal decision whether you use these methods to reduce stress and balance your bodily functions. As with any new technique or program, talk with your doctor to determine what makes sense for you.

CHAPTER FIVE

for men only

As you daydream and plan on becoming a dad, you never think about infertility until the stun of it knocks you to your knees. Infertility, although a shock to you as an individual, is not an uncommon condition for the male partner. In fact, male infertility is just as likely as female infertility in a couple's inability to conceive.

Assumptions

Before Brian and I tied the knot, our conversations were rare regarding when to have children. We didn't think there was much to discuss, because we assumed we had all the time in the world. We focused on traveling around the United States and other countries, like Italy, Turkey, and Greece. We took our time when it came to making babies.

I'd always wanted kids and just assumed that I'd have children in the future with my wife, but it wasn't a lifelong goal for me. I thought it would just happen naturally one day. When we got married, Lesley and I were on the same page, knowing we wanted to start a family. I never thought there would be a problem.

The whole time I was assuming that kids would come along for Lesley and me. It got to the point where Lesley was not getting pregnant, but I wasn't freaked out about it. Lesley had a stressful job that threw a wrench into trying to have kids. I thought that if she got into a slower-paced job things would be okay.

Finally, Lesley changed jobs and we moved to a family-friendly town to could focus on having kids. We bought a house within walking distance of one of the best elementary schools in the county. Lesley had a home office working as a freelance writer and I was five miles from work. We structured our lives for kids.

Sometimes I think that if I were more passionate about having children, I probably would not have been so laid back about making it happen. I wanted kids and thought it would be great to have them. I just never thought we would have difficulty.

~ Brian

Men and Emotions

When a reproductive problem occurs, it seems that most doctors and nurses focus all of their attention on the woman. While men are very much a part of the equation, they are limited to just standing on the sidelines during pelvic exams and ultrasounds. Because of all the drama, women sometimes fail to remember that their men feel devastated, just as they do.

Often it's extremely difficult for men to express their feelings. Further, we forget that men have feelings at all, simply because they don't reveal their emotions. To make matters worse, our culture stereotypes men by venerating the "strong silent types" in movies and TV shows. It's a lot of pressure for any man to endure.

Most men don't know how to express their feelings because they've never been given permission to show emotions. They were taught to hide their feelings, that tears are a sign of weakness. They certainly aren't comfortable showing fear or being indecisive. Many men believe their role is to be a provider for their families, taking care of everyone's well-being. Men want to fix things and situations. If they can't find a solution for problems, they may get discouraged and frustrated. When dealing with infertility, men often feel deeply frustrated because there are no clear-cut solutions or answers. For many men, the emotion that's likely to surface is anger over their frustration. Anger is the emotion society allows men to reveal. It's considered to be a man's "right" or a sign of his virility.

When most men see their partners in emotional or physical pain, they want to make things better. When infertility affects a man's ability to create a family, he may feel inadequate or powerless. His ability to procreate, the most basic and natural drive he knows, is taken away. And despite the fact that anger is the emotion that comes to the surface, most men feel sad and disappointed, because their personal expectations of having children are not being met.

Pregnancy loss and fertility problems affect men the same way they affect women. Men, like women, feel discouraged, powerless, and confused. Fertility problems are difficult to experience. It's also challenging to understand the medical terminology.

Men need time to process the new information they hear, and they may want space. A few men may want to sit and talk for hours on end about their feelings, but women shouldn't expect it. Some men like to process their thoughts and feelings by tinkering in the garage; others escape by watching football or baseball. Every guy is different. The women in their lives should try to be sensitive to their needs and allow them to cope in their unique way.

It's About Him

I have a tendency to get caught up in my own emotions and sometimes forget that my husband needs me. One day I was sitting on the sofa with Brian, feeling depressed and sad about my inability to have children. I was crying and talking, feeling overwhelmed by my own thoughts and feelings. As I reached for a tissue on the coffee table, I looked over at Brian and saw something in his eyes that made me stop and think. *'Oh my God, he's really hurting, too, right now, and here I am crying and blubbering about my feelings. He's not saying much. I need to shut up and give him room to talk and even cry if he feels like it. I should be comforting him.'*

I quickly wiped my nose and then wrapped my arms around his broad shoulders. Kissing his cheek I said, "Honey, I know I've been rattling on, but it's not all about me. I'm here for you. I understand that you are hurting. You have emotions and need to be heard, too. Know that I'm here for you. Please let me be strong for you, just like you've been strong for me. I love you."

He bowed his head and tears started dropping from his eyes. I felt his big shoulders quake beneath my arms. I was so thankful that I'd realized he needed my support and that I was able to comfort him. I prayed silently, God, help me be strong for him. Help us get through this together. Amen.

The Male Infertility Factor

Infertility affects both women and men about 50-50. In almost half the cases, infertility is a male problem that needs to be investigated through sperm and blood tests. Increasingly, men are scheduling appointments with urologists and fertility specialists to solve their own reproductive challenges. It's no longer assumed that failure to reproduce is entirely a woman's issue, but sometimes it's still difficult for men to come to terms with their own situation.

Luckily for me, Brian was open-minded and willing to meet with reproductive specialists. He was just as intent as I was on knowing why we couldn't easily get pregnant.

> *Lesley had already had two ectopic pregnancies, when her OB-GYN suggested we look into other options for having children. The doctor referred us to a fertility specialist who asked me to submit my sperm for analysis. I didn't think our "problem" was a sperm issue. I thought the problem was just Lesley's one blocked tube.*
>
> *Honestly, it didn't offend me and I thought I might as well get my sperm checked. I figured we needed to explore all of our options, but I really didn't expect the doctors to find anything wrong with me.*
>
> *I told them, "Fine, test my sperm."*
>
> *Except for a few embarrassing moments, it wasn't a big deal.*
>
> **~ Brian**

One of the most common causes of male infertility is low sperm count. Since it only takes one special little sperm to fertilize an egg, it doesn't seem like it would be a big deal. Right? Well, it's complicated. The vagina presents many obstacles to the hundreds of sperm hoping to swim their way to the finish line. Sperm must survive in the vagina's acidic environment with a 4.2 pH. Interestingly enough, to help sperm survive, semen changes the pH to 7.2.

Sperm must also cross the "Great Barrier Reef," aka cervical mucus, which by design is thick to keep sperm out of the uterus. It's as if a "Do Not Enter" sign is posted, discouraging sperm from trespassing. The only time the mucus changes is right before ovulation, when it becomes thin and slippery, like raw egg whites. During this small window of opportunity, sperm are actually encouraged to pass through the cervix, entering the uterus in search of their target: the egg.

Finally, sperm must swim through the fallopian tubes to find the egg. They have no idea which tube contains the egg. Some will swim into the wrong tube and be out of luck. Others will choose the correct tube and find what they're looking for.

"Only a few hundred sperm will actually swim up to the fallopian tubes," according to Endocrinologist and Fertility Expert Dr. Lori Arnold, Scientific Director of La Jolla IVF in La Jolla, California. Therefore, having a low sperm count decreases your chance of getting your partner pregnant, because the odds of a single sperm reaching the egg are very low.

What is a Semen Analysis?

A semen analysis is the basic test to determine a man's fertility. If the semen does not contain sperm, your efforts to conceive will be in vain. The best part about it is that a semen analysis is painless. Dr. Kettel said Brian's semen sample would be checked for any abnormalities and give us information on number of sperm in the sample (count), the amount of sperm produced (volume), the number of sperm per milliliter (concentration), how well the sperm move around (motility), and the shape of the sperm (morphology).

Most men ejaculate about one-half to one teaspoon of semen, and the color of the semen should be a whitish-gray. Men are diagnosed with infertility if their count is lower than 20 million per milliliter of semen.

It was important for us to know about Brian's sperm motility and morphology because we wanted to try to predict our potential success with IVF. We also needed to determine whether I would be a candidate for intracytoplasmic sperm injection (ICSI), if needed. (As previously mentioned, ICSI is a method of injecting sperm with poor motility directly into the egg.) Thus, Dr. Kettel could ensure success of egg penetration by the sperm, increasing a successful outcome for us.

> It took a couple of days for the semen tests to be finished. The doctor called us into his office to discuss my results.
>
> I was surprised to hear Dr. Kettel tell us that I had low-quality semen. He said I had low sperm count, poor morphology, and poor motility. None of the results were ideal.
>
> Knowing we could use ICSI to overcome my sperm's poor motility gave us some hope, but we would have to roll the dice with my morphology. I couldn't do much about that. The news certainly didn't make me feel good.
>
> Getting my sperm test results back explained why Lesley and I had experienced such a hard time getting pregnant in the first place. We knew she only had one good fallopian tube, and now we knew that the quality of my sperm wasn't good. I was disappointed to see that we both had fertility issues. That meant our odds were even less than I thought they were.
>
> **~ Brian**

Physical Exam

After the sperm tests, Brian had to get a physical. I sat in the exam room while the urologist, who was a fertility specialist, performed the evaluation. Surprisingly, the exam didn't take very long. The doctor checks for any abnormalities, such as large varicoceles, undescended testes, absence of vasa deferentia (tubes that transport sperm), or cysts. The doctor explained to us that varicoceles are the veins that drain the testicles in the scrotum. He said they feel "like a bag of worms." Luckily, Brian's worms were just fine.

The doctor also said smaller-sized and softer testicles are sometimes evidence of low sperm count and may show problems with sperm formation.

Fortunately, Brian received a clean bill of health.

Overcoming Male Infertility

The urologist gave Brian several suggestions to help increase his overall health and fertility. Smoking damages sperm DNA. But Brian doesn't smoke, so we didn't have to worry about that. Here are the doctor's recommendations:

- Avoid hot tubs or whirlpool baths.

- Eat a fiber-rich diet, including fresh vegetables, beans, and peas.

- Avoid eating processed foods from boxes or plastic packaging.

- Avoid foods with fatty animal products (e.g., fried foods, donuts, and cookies).

- Stay away from foods containing estrogen (e.g., beef from hormone-fed cows).

- Avoid dairy products from hormone-fed cows.

- Take a daily vitamin supplement with vitamin C and E, selenium, beta carotene and zinc.

- Wear cotton boxers and stay away from G-strings with synthetic fabrics.

• Avoid contact with heavy metals (mercury and lead).

Causes of Low Sperm Count

Low sperm count may be attributed to causes such as trauma to the testicles, hormonal imbalances, infections, blocked vasa deferentia, chemotherapy, genetic problems, and mumps. In addition to swallowing vitamins, eating fiber-rich diets, and banning hot tubs, IUI and IVF can also help couples produce a pregnancy when low sperm count threatens their ability to start a family.

> *About 85 to 90 percent of all male infertility problems are attributed to low sperm count and poor sperm quality. Additionally, the sperm may have poor morphology and function abnormally, failing to properly fertilize the egg. A few men have no sperm at all, but those cases account for less than 5 percent of male infertility.*
>
> **~ Dr. Kettel**

Jim's Story: Sperm Retrieval

When there's no sperm in a man's ejaculate, the sperm can be surgically removed from his testicles or epididymis (the beginning of the vas deferens). There are several outpatient procedures for sperm retrieval. Jim learned first-hand how simple the procedure could be when he made an appointment with a urologist. He and his wife had been trying to start their family for seven years without any success.

> *I always thought something was wrong with Monica, but after years of her not getting pregnant I agreed to get checked out by a urologist. I found out that I was missing a tube called the vas deferens. It's a tube that transports the sperm. Mine couldn't*

get out. The urologist gave me a local anesthetic and took my sperm out of my testicles and froze them so we could do IVF later.

On Monica's third IVF cycle using my frozen sperm, she got pregnant. We were surprised and relieved. We could never have had our baby without my having the sperm procedure.

~ Jim

Ted and Emily's Story: Electroejaculation

Few men are willing to admit that they cannot ejaculate. It's a highly personal and private matter. It's also a medical condition. The inability to ejaculate is most commonly caused by spinal cord injury. An estimated 10,000 cases occur each year in the United States. Other causes include high blood pressure medications, testicular injury, chemotherapy, blockage in the reproductive system, sexually transmitted diseases, cystic fibrosis, hormone deficiencies, and kidney disease.[9]

Emily and Ted met in college and eventually married. During the first ten years of their relationship they tried not to get pregnant. When it was time to have children, things weren't working out as they planned. Emily shares their story.

Ted injured his spinal cord during college, when he was on the swim team. Luckily his accident didn't paralyze him, but he has suffered from neck and back problems ever since. The thing he didn't know until we tried to get pregnant is that the injury affected his fertility. He can't always ejaculate, and tests showed that his sperm production was low. I know it bugs him. He makes jokes about it, saying stuff like, "I wish I could shoot like a porn star."

We went to a male infertility specialist who told us about electroejaculation. Ted actually knew what it was, since his dad is in the cattle breeding business. He had watched veterinarians test his dad's prize bulls' sperm, so he knew exactly what it entailed.

The thing the doctor used looked very similar to a smaller version of a cattle prod. The doctor removed Ted's sperm and froze them. As soon as we save up enough money we're going to do IVF and, hopefully, we'll have twins.

~ Emily

Electroejaculation only takes about thirty minutes for the procedure. The man lies on his side and is typically given a general anesthesia. First, the doctor examines his rectum to make sure there are no obstructions, such as polyps. Next, a probe, which is attached to electrical currents, is inserted into the anus. To accommodate each individual, the doctor manually adjusts the electrical pulses to stimulate an erection and ejaculation. The sperm is collected and stored for later use.

Infertility Affects Marriages

I have an acquaintance whose husband divorced her after she couldn't bear his children. He eventually found a younger wife who was fertile as a rabbit. Another friend divorced her husband because he wouldn't agree to do IVF. She was desperate to have a baby and ended up using a sperm donor. Today, she is raising twins as a single mom. Other marriages fall apart because of resentments and wounds that are too deep to heal. Some stick it out and grow stronger in their relationship because of the shared life crisis. Everyone deals with stress and infertility in very different ways.

When it's difficult to communicate with your significant other, how do you bridge the gap of silence? What do you say when words seem out of reach? How can you help one another heal and get beyond the pain of unmet expectations and broken dreams?

Often, words are inadequate and silence is the only thing you can share. During those times, let sleeping dogs lie. Be quiet.

Hold hands. Sit next to each other. Breathe. Take a walk together. Just be. Being present for each other is enough most of the time. When you want to comfort your significant other, try using words of affirmation such as:

- I'm so glad we have each other.

- Honey (or your term of endearment), I have no idea what you are feeling but I want you to know that I love you.

- If you need me, I am here for you.

- You mean the world to me.

- Let me know if you need a shoulder to lean on.

- We're going to get through this together.

Questions to Stimulate Conversation

Don't let emotional and mental stress distance you and your significant other for too long. Find ways to celebrate your relationship and focus on the positive aspects of your life together. When you're ready to open up and talk, here are some key questions to help the two of you connect:

- What are you thinking right now?

- How do you feel?

- What has been the toughest challenge for you?

- How can I best support you?

- Where would you like to vacation this coming year?

Different Viewpoints

I wish I could compartmentalize my feelings like Brian. It would make life so much easier. Brian and I have handled our fertility problems differently. Brian is able to box up his feelings, not allowing them to spill over into his day-to-day activities.

Whether or not I have children infiltrates my every thought

and future plans. For example, when I recently joined a new reading group, I had to choose between the "young mothers" or "career-minded" group. That one choice alone threw the entire fertility drama into my face. My going back to school for a PhD all depends on whether or not we're going to do IVF again. We live in a house with four bedrooms. But, we might as well move back into a small condo, since we don't have children.

In my mind, our fertility affects everything. Brian sees our fertility problems as just that—a problem—something that he doesn't think about when at work or on the basketball court or on vacation. I admire his ability to segregate his thoughts.

When Brian and I did IVF, we were hopeful that the procedure would give us a baby. Once we transitioned from our fertility doctor to my OB-GYN, we thought it would be smooth sailing. When our fetus's heartbeat stopped and I had to be the bearer of bad news to Brian, he demonstrated his ability to compartmentalize his feelings even when our hopes and dreams were shattered.

> *I was sitting in class when I got a text message from Lesley. I figured she was letting me know that she was done at her ultrasound appointment.*
>
> *Now, with our third pregnancy, I was in a heightened state of alert, but I was growing more and more excited about the new addition to our lives. I was thrilled about the joy and challenges a baby was going to bring.*
>
> *In our third pregnancy, we bypassed Lesley's bad fallopian tube by using IVF to deposit the fertilized egg directly into her womb. Most importantly, the embryo implanted into her uterus and we'd seen our fetus's beating heart multiple times. That was a first. We never saw a heartbeat with Lesley's first two pregnancies.*
>
> *With a "mission accomplished" grin, our fertility doctor assured us that the tough part was over. He said we had a 95 percent chance of having a live birth. I felt we were free and clear of the past problems, so I had finally let my guard down a little.*
>
> *Glancing at Lesley's text, my heart skipped a beat. It read, "Call me ASAP...urgent."*

For a moment, I remembered the previous day in class when our professor started the day with an icebreaker. He asked all the students to share something about themselves that nobody else knew. We went around the room listening to tales of previous stints in rock bands, stories of obscure hobbies, reports of drinking specialty coffee produced by beans excreted from a wildcat, and other crazy stories. I was sitting in the back of the class, so I had time to decide that this would be the moment to share my good news—I was going to be a dad for the first time.

The guy next to me took his turn. He was at least 10 years my junior. He spoke up and said, "My wife's pregnant and we're going to have our first child!" The class applauded. Then, it was my turn.

Looking at the guy next to me I said, "You took mine!"

I repeated his news and the class applauded once again.

Thinking back, the words I said that day, "You took mine," were very prophetic.

Again, I looked down at Lesley's text, trying to convince myself that it wasn't a big deal. I read it again. "Call me ASAP...urgent."

I quietly slipped out of the lecture hall and walked out of the building into a glorious San Diego day, with clear blue skies overhead and a slight ocean breeze. I speed-dialed Lesley.

"Hello," Lesley answered.

I tried to sound casual even though I felt tense. "What's up, honey?"

She didn't say anything and I knew she was crying. Barely audible through the tears, she explained, "The ultrasound. There's no heartbeat." Then she started sobbing uncontrollably.

I was speechless as I stared at the pink flowers blooming along the sidewalk. Everything was silent around me, except for birds singing nearby, enjoying their beautiful spring day.

I remember thinking sarcastically, Thank you God for blessing me so. This is the answer to my prayers. Thanks so much.

Then my thoughts turned back to Lesley and the agony I knew she was feeling.

"Where are you? I'll be there right away."

I returned to class, packed up my books and left. I knew that my own grief could wait. Class could definitely wait. Now, it was time to be the comforter.

~ Brian

Suggested Questions for Couples to Consider

Answering the following questions before beginning ART can provide guidelines that will help you maintain perspective:

- Are we going to discuss our fertility issues with family and friends?

- How many cycles of ART will we try?

- What are our emotional, physical, and financial limits?

- How "far" are we willing to go to have a baby (e.g., borrowing money from family, getting a second mortgage, draining retirements accounts, etc.)?

- What is most important to us individually and collectively (e.g., staying sane, keeping our marriage healthy, pursuing a career, etc.)?

- How will we handle disagreements regarding our reproductive abilities, limits, and desires?

CHAPTER SIX

dealing with grief

No one ever told me that grief felt so like fear.
At other times it feels like being mildly drunk, or
confused. There is a sort of invisible blanket between
the world and me. I find it hard to take in what
anyone says. Or perhaps, hard to want to take it in.
~ C.S. Lewis, A Grief Observed

Infertility constitutes a loss—the loss of a dream to bear your own child. When faced with this condition, you grieve by alternately entertaining denial, anger, bargaining attempts, and depression as you attempt to make sense of your struggle. The journey is all yours to advance and retreat—in and out of the steps—as best suits your needs. Elisabeth Kubler-Ross explains the grieving process in depth in her book, *On Death and Dying*. None of the steps are mandatory but they do offer a clear road map for your recovery. Become acquainted with grief's many faces as you find strength to cope with your very deep and personal loss.

It's hard to mourn for my baby when I never had
the chance to hold it's little body in my arms. But I
still feel a sense of loss and sadness that's hard to put
into words.

~ Sarah

119

Support Systems

Where do you find solace? Within yourself? Through friends and family? Staying busy with work or social activities? When you face challenges such as pregnancy loss or infertility, it is very important to have an emotional support system. There are many ways to create emotional support systems for yourself, such as counseling, positive psychology, maintaining a "can do" attitude, and mindfulness.

I have utilized each one of these support systems in my journey through pregnancy loss and infertility. I have also found support through meditation and through prayer, calling on my Higher Power, aka God. All of these resources have helped me deal with my interior pain and struggle.

Where do you find inner strength? You may or may not believe in God. I am not here to judge, only to offer words of encouragement and support. Praying to God is valuable to me because it gives me a place to put my anger. I do not want to project my rage onto my husband, friends, or family. They don't deserve to suffer just because I'm in pain. The truth is that they probably couldn't handle my anger. It would hurt my relationship with them, but I can scream at God. I believe God can take it. So, when I speak of God in the following pages, feel free to insert the name of your Higher Power wherever I mention God. My goal is to offer suggestions, ideas for support systems, and resources to help you move forward in healthy and meaningful ways. Adapt them to suit your own beliefs and situation.

Shocking Grief

My first encounter with grief was at the tender age of eight. My father, while crop dusting, crashed his plane. He died instantly in the crumbled wreckage. The FAA investigated the crash site but never determined a cause for the accident. It could have been a gust of wind, mechanical failure, or just pilot's error. No one will ever know. The only eyewitness was a local farmer who watched the plane go down. Dad's face and body were mangled from the crash, so he had a closed casket during the visitation and funeral. I never had the chance to say goodbye.

The meaning of Dad's death didn't actually sink in until six months later. My little terrier-mix dog was hit by a car. A neighbor brought Candy to me in a small box. Her white-, black-, and brown-spotted coat was tangled in blood. Overwhelmed by my sense of loss, I cried uncontrollably. Seeing my beloved dog lying in a box reminded me of the big box in which my dad had been laid to rest.

Experiencing two profound losses at an early age taught me not to expect everything in life to work out. I quit believing in fairy-tale endings.

Then I met Brian and fell hopelessly in love. Once we were married and settled into our new life together, I thought things would be different. With the promise of our happy marriage I allowed myself to dream again, and that included having a family of our own with two or three children.

Denial

After my first pregnancy loss I experienced denial. I refused to believe it could happen again. A year later my doctor diagnosed me with a second tubal pregnancy. At that point I had to face the reality of two losses.

Then, when my third pregnancy loss occurred because of a miscarriage, I moved from denial into a state of shock. I felt traumatized. The accumulation of my losses and compounded grief made me feel as if I had no control over my life.

> *Experiencing a pregnancy loss is very traumatic. It's a complex grief because everything is backwards. Instead of having a lifetime of memories, as you do when you lose a loved one later in life, there is no storehouse of memories. When a baby has been lost, often the only memories one has are traumatic, and it's very difficult. Whatever you feel during the*

process, such as sadness, grief, anger, and fear, is normal.

A perinatal loss so difficult, because miscarriage is often considered, medically speaking, not an uncommon event. The medical staff and other caring people don't often realize what's been lost. They say, 'Don't worry, you can have another baby.' They say things like this rather than being able to acknowledge that this couple has lost their child.

~ Dr. Martha Diamond, co-founder of Center for Reproductive Psychology and co-author of *Unsung Lullabies: Understanding and Coping with Infertility*

Painful Grief

Experiencing grief is something we all share, because we all suffer loss in one way or another. We grieve from loss throughout our lives: a broken toy, a best friend moving, the death of a loved one, divorce, and traumatic experiences, such as a pregnancy loss and infertility. Every loss has a unique impact.

The feelings that are associated with grief include anger, anxiety, guilt, sadness, and loneliness. You may also feel worthless, thinking you have failed in comparison to childbearing friends. You may be irritable because you are frustrated by the unknown. You may ache with an emptiness that only a child can fill and feel pained by jealousy over other families with children. All of these feelings are normal. They are part of the grieving process.

My first tubal pregnancy occurred at eight weeks and six days. I was upset because the loss seemed pointless. My fetus didn't have a chance to grow. I felt cheated out of the promise of a new life. My entire body ached from grief. I experienced severe backaches, daily migraines, and insomnia from the stress and grief I suffered. I was low spirited and sad. Food had never been a vice for me, but in my deep anguish I turned to Southern comfort dishes from my childhood. For the first time, I began overeating. I ate to try to fill my void.

For months I lost all interest in work, playing tennis, or seeing friends. I cried whenever I saw other women with babies. Just the sight of children made me ache in the pit of my stomach. I stopped going to church. I couldn't watch movies about families, death, or dying. Commercials with babies made me sob. I felt like a failure. It was difficult to be happy for my pregnant friends. I even skipped a few baby showers without sending gifts, because I couldn't handle the confrontation.

I was mourning a deep loss and felt completely hopeless. I also felt like no one understood my pain except my husband. So, I didn't really want to talk about it with anyone. I wanted to crawl under the covers and stay there. Some days I even wanted to die.

That's what grief does to you.

Angry Grief

After I recovered from the laparoscopic surgery of my first tubal pregnancy, my emotional and physical pain turned into anger. Every time I went to the bathroom, showered, or changed my clothes, I saw my abdominal scars where the doctor had made the three small incisions to remove my fetus. The scars reminded me of the little baby I lost. I felt ashamed that I couldn't bring a child into the world. Looking at my scars I wondered what was wrong with me.

Honestly, I wanted to blame someone else for my pain and anger, but I couldn't point a finger. No one was to blame, not even God. Nevertheless, I was angry with God because I believed God had the ability to bless me with a child. From where I sat, it appeared as if God was ignoring me, so I decided to give God the silent treatment. I quit praying for a while. My spiritual life suffered, and I felt a void because of the distance I'd put between me and God.

Eventually I realized that I was being childish. I considered reasons beyond my understanding regarding why my ectopic may have occurred. Maybe the baby would have been mentally or physically handicapped in some horrible way. Maybe I was being spared from having to make difficult decisions.

Random thoughts ran through my mind. I wanted to pinpoint a reason why it happened. After dreaming up every imaginable cause, I finally chalked it up as a fluke, just like my dad's plane crash. I figured it was a random act of nature. That was the only thing that made sense to me.

Despite my attempts to make sense out of my loss, the grief wouldn't let go of me. I knew there was no escaping or running from it, so I was determined to face it head on and let it wash over me like waves slamming upon the beach.

Whenever I get confused, I write poems to assign words to my mixed-up feelings. The following poem was born out of the dark despair of my muddled mind.

I'm on a ship sinking slowly
The shore is in sight
Though sunshine surrounds me
The wind blows coldly
Will I make it to the water's edge?
Or will I disappear into the ocean's depth?
No one knows
Control cannot be had
I am helplessly waiting
To glimpse my fate

While I was drifting deeper into a bottomless pit of despair, I started seeing little glimpses of hope. Friends would say kind words. My husband would be extra sweet to me on days when I felt really sad. I felt their love holding me up and surrounding me. It was a difficult time, but the love of family and friends helped me weather the storm.

Kim's Story: Bitter Grief

Kim experienced four failed IVF cycles. She and her husband, Jeffrey, lost hope and became very bitter about having children. She couldn't understand why IVF had worked for her sister and best friend but not for her. Kim talks about her feelings of grief.

My inability to have children made me question my faith. I thought "What did I do to deserve this?" I was angry and wondered why everyone else could get pregnant but not me. For a long time I was very bitter. Every time I flipped through a People Magazine and saw pregnant celebrities, I sarcastically thought to myself, "Of course she's having a baby. She's beautiful and has millions of dollars. Life is picture perfect for her. Of course she's pregnant."

It looked so easy for everyone around me. My best friend got pregnant when she was 41 and again at 43. It just wasn't fair.

My brother-in-law's sister, who is 45, is pregnant with their fifth child. She "accidentally" got pregnant and now they're worrying the baby will have Down Syndrome. They are scared, but I am jealous.

When I compare my situation to other women who have had babies, I realize that fertility is not fair. There is no fairness when it comes to fertility. You could be a hateful person and still be very fertile.

Being infertile has opened my eyes, making me realize that I can't have everything I want. I may never be able to share in the joys of having a family with my husband. That saddens me, but I'm learning to be content with what I have: a wonderful guy who really loves me. We have a really good marriage, and that is a good thing. Not everyone has what we have.

~ Kim

Depressed Grief

When Brian and I originally decided to have children, I was ready to switch gears from career mode to being his baby-mama. I was proud of the fact that we were going to create a family together. My plan was to be a stay-at-home-mom who baked cookies, scheduled play dates, managed the household, and greeted her husband with a kiss after work each day. I also planned to start writing novels in between diaper changes.

After my pregnancy losses, I was mentally wiped out and felt discouraged about the future. I lost my zest for life and vision for work. Every ounce of ambition vanished and I had no desire to create new goals. Feeling I had nothing to live for, I wanted to sleep my life away. My grandfather's voice echoed in my head saying, "Lesley, you're gonna sleep your life away. You better get up." He'd said those words to me when I was a little girl. Grandfather's voice was crystal clear to me in the darkness. His words were my only motivation to get out of bed each day.

I've heard it said that when you lose a parent, you've lost your past. When you lose your spouse, you've lost your present. When you lose your child, you've lost your future.

Jessica and Andrew's Story: Questioning Grief

Jessica, 35, and Andrew, 37, already had two healthy children, a 7-year-old daughter and a 5-year-old son. They were a happy family, yet longed for even more kids. They knew children were a big responsibility, but enjoyed the rigors of parenting.

When they tried to have more children, things didn't go as planned. Jessica and Andrew experienced a grief they'd never known before. By sharing her story, Jessica hopes to help other couples who have suffered a similar loss.

With my first two pregnancies I didn't have any
trouble but, from the beginning of my third pregnancy,
I knew something was wrong. My hormone levels
were okay and the doctor said everything looked good,

but I wasn't having typical pregnancy symptoms, like nausea. That was a big red flag for me, because I was really sick with my first two pregnancies.

During my eighth-week ultrasound, the doctor said my fetus's size was a little off, but he assured me that everything was fine. My hormone levels continued to rise until eleven weeks, when I started bleeding. I went in for an ultrasound and there was no heartbeat. The doctor wanted to do a D&C. But I wasn't ready to make that decision. I went home and planned to go back to his office with my decision the next day.

That night I started bleeding and having really bad cramps. After about six hours I felt a gush come out. I thought it would be blood, so I went to the bathroom to change my underwear and pad. When I pulled down my pants and sat on the commode, I looked down and saw my baby's head on the pad.

In hindsight, I think the cramping and pain that I felt were timed contractions, just like you have with labor. At the time I didn't realize it. I think the gush that I felt was my water breaking, and that's when our baby came out. A few minutes later, the afterbirth came out just like it did when I had my daughter and my son.

It was very traumatic seeing the little head of our baby. We could see her ears starting to form and her little mouth. We could see the tongue starting to form in her mouth. It was perfectly formed. I don't know what happened to her body. It probably just went down the toilet as I was sitting there.

My husband and I were devastated over the loss of our baby. It put us in an awkward position, wondering what to do. We weren't just gonna flush our baby's head down the toilet like a piece of trash.

So, we chose to bury her in a small case. We named her Hope and buried her at a cemetery where my family had a plot.

I was upset about how my pregnancy ended. It was a double-edged sword, meaning I was grateful that I got to see my baby's face. That was all I was every gonna have or see but, then again, seeing her made it so much more painful and more real.

I questioned God and asked why it happened. I don't understand why God allows miscarriages to happen. It's such an unnecessary pain to have to endure. It seemed so senseless to me. I kept wondering, Why did God put us through that? I would rather not have gotten pregnant at all.

I was angry about the whole thing and directed my anger at Andrew, because he never listened when I told him that something was wrong with my pregnancy. It put a strain on our marriage. He kept parroting the doctors, saying, "Everything is fine and your hormone levels are good." It was a real struggle between us. I was mad and frustrated at my husband because he didn't believe me. After we lost the baby I was angry at him because I felt like he hadn't supported me and believed me. When the miscarriage happened, I told him, "See, I told you something was wrong and you just kept believing the doctors."

After my miscarriage I also told Andrew, "In the future you need to trust me and not be dismissive of what I'm telling you. I'm not one to exaggerate. Everyone was ignoring me when I said something was wrong with my pregnancy. I need you on my side."

I guess it's natural for everyone to believe the doctors since they are the experts. My husband has always been that way, believing anything a doctor says. I always listen to my body and question things when it doesn't seem right.

Doctors should listen to their patients and not dismiss everything they say. Doctors shouldn't rely just on ultrasounds and hormone tests. Women know their bodies.

Six months later I got pregnant again. Early on, I knew something was wrong and at thirteen weeks I miscarried. The doctor wanted to do a D&C, but I felt it was too invasive. He said I might hemorrhage, which could be dangerous.

Once again I decided to go home. Just like before, I started cramping and having contractions. I got scared and decided to let the doctors do a D&C, because I didn't want my baby's body flushed down the toilet again. We hurried to the emergency room. Right after the nurses settled me into a room, I felt a gush of water, just like before, and the baby's body came out. I could even feel the baby's little legs and arms as I delivered him.

The nurse scooped my baby's body up and put him in a container. We told the doctors and nurses that we wanted genetic testing done to determine what went wrong. We were very clear about our intentions and they assured us that testing would be done. I was drugged up because I was in so much pain and trusted Andrew to make sure our wishes were carried out.

Later that night we went home. Andrew woke me up saying that the hospital screwed up by putting our baby in formaldehyde. That meant they couldn't do genetic testing. Formaldehyde prevents them from growing the tissue to try and find abnormalities in the tissue. Now, we'd never know what went wrong with our baby. It flipped me out. I was furious and upset that we never got to see him. I felt so guilty. I wondered if I made the right decision to go to the ER. After everything that we went through, we got nothing out of it. I was so angry.

We went to the hospital to pick up our baby's body. I was so pissed because the doctors had put our baby in formaldehyde, and because of the expense of another funeral. It had been a bad year for us financially. We never could have anticipated the burden of funeral costs for two babies.

The funeral home typically only buried stillbirth babies, so they didn't even know how to deal with us. When a baby is under twenty weeks, you can basically do whatever you want. You can bury the baby in your backyard if you want. That made me feel sad. The lives of our babies were minimized because of their gestational ages. It angered me, too. If people could see what we saw—our baby's face, arms, and legs—our two babies were human.

I sobbed when I read the pathologist report declaring that our baby was a boy. When I looked at him, he was beautiful and perfect. That made me more angry, and this time I was angry at God, wondering what had gone wrong. It looked like there was nothing wrong with our son. I almost wanted there to be something wrong with him, just so we could have an answer as to why it happened. To see our perfectly formed little baby at thirteen weeks was heartbreaking and upsetting. I struggled a lot and I'm still struggling with my anger about the two failed pregnancies.

I'm not sure if I should try to have another baby. My desire to have a child far outweighs my fear of having another miscarriage, but my husband is having second thoughts. He thinks we should just be thankful for the two children we have and be content. We're struggling even more now because we're in disagreement. He's afraid because, if we get pregnant again, he doesn't know where it will take me emotionally.

~ **Jessica**

Jessica finally got her happy ending. One year after her second miscarriage she conceived once again. Only this time Jessica enjoyed a healthy, full-term pregnancy and delivered a baby boy. She and Andrew named him Benjamin, after his great-grandfather.

Steps to Help You Deal with Grief

We live in a culture that expects us to just get over it. Mourn quickly and get back to work and life. It's hard to mourn when everyone around you is uncomfortable with your grief. People usually don't know what to say to someone who has experienced infertility or the loss of a baby. Some people don't even think you should grieve the death of an eight-week-old fetus. People who have not had similar experiences may find it hard to empathize.

When I was doing IVF, I never told anyone at work that I was trying to have a baby. I didn't want to deal with their constant questions and their wondering eyes looking at my belly. I also knew I didn't want to hear "I'm sorry" from a hundred different people if my IVF procedure didn't work.

When we experience reproductive challenges like ectopic pregnancies, miscarriages, and stillbirths, emotions such as fear, anger, and grief often arise. To enjoy a truly fulfilling and meaningful life, we must let go of those emotions, because toxic thinking and negative feelings will only leave us bitter.

So, how do you quit living in fear? When you're angry at the world because your expectations are not being met, how do you let go of the rage? When your heart is broken, how do you manage your grief?

Time

Take time to move through your fear, anger, and grief. The process cannot be forced or hurried. It can take months and even years. The amount of time needed to process those negative emotions is different for each person. Such feelings are highly personal experiences and hard to communicate. Some people worry, thinking they should have gotten over a divorce, pregnancy loss, or the death of a pet more quickly than they do. They think something is wrong with them when they still feel anger or sadness after six months. There is no timetable. It's a process.

Have a Good Cry

Tears help us heal by releasing the pent-up emotions of anger, fear, sorrow, and disappointment. After a good cry, most people feel an overall sense of well-being, because tears release toxins from our bodies that are caused by stress (7). When it comes to grief and loss, tears are very beneficial.

After my IVF cycle ended in a miscarriage, I woke up from the D&C feeling overwhelmed by sadness, knowing I had lost another baby. I sobbed because my baby was gone and I'd never get to see her or hold her. I experienced compounded grief, because it was my third pregnancy loss. The trauma was far too deep to hide. My pain was profound.

Lying on the recovery table, my body felt weak and heavy, because I was under the influence of anesthesia. The lights in the room were almost blinding and the bed was lumpy. Tubes poked out of my arms and monitors were attached to my chest. I heard a beeping sound next to my bed. My heartbeat. I cried even harder. I wanted to hear my baby's heartbeat. My brother Chris stood at my bedside. As I sobbed uncontrollably, he put his arms around me and said, "I'm here. Cry all you want. You're gonna get through this."

Talk It Out

If you can find a good friend who's willing to listen as you talk about your loss, it will help you heal. Loss can make you feel completely alone and isolated from others. Talking about your thoughts and feelings makes the journey more bearable.

Consider the Source

Most people are uncomfortable with grief and certainly don't know how to handle another person's anguish. Their inappropriate words may stem from lack of experience. Most have never dealt with a pregnancy loss or infertility problems. Put the best spin possible on other people's comments.

Find a Support Group

Seek out people who will be comforting and encouraging. The best people to surround yourself with during times of grief are people who have had similar experiences. The National Infertility Association, also known as RESOLVE, has support groups around the country for men and women struggling with fertility issues. Invite family and friends to the support group to help them better understand what you're going through, or offer them information on infertility and pregnancy loss.

Ask for Help

If you're feeling emotionally and physically drained, ask for help. Lean on your family and friends during this time. Ask them for assistance with tasks that may feel too overwhelming, such as shopping for groceries, laundry, or car repairs.

Take a Trip

Give yourself a break. Don't minimize your feelings and think you should be getting over your grief quickly. If you have the ability to go on a trip, then do it. Even if you cannot afford a vacation, take a drive along a different route. Go on a day-trip to a neighboring city or town. Change your scenery. Going to an unfamiliar place will remind you that there are new adventures waiting for you.

Know Your Limits

It's normal not to feel comfortable with other moms. Don't feel obligated to attend baby showers or children's birthday parties. Let friends and family know that it's a difficult time for you, and you wish them well, but that you need time away right now. When responding to invitations, know and set your limits. Be kind to yourself first.

Realize that, during holidays and anniversaries, you and your significant other may feel sadder than usual. It's normal. When special days arrive, you may feel a wave of sorrow because you are reminded of your loss. Consider staying home if you are still grieving, or set limits on events you choose to attend.

At some point you will feel less weighed down by your grief. You may not have all the answers, but you will be ready to move forward. In the meantime, just take one day, and if needed one hour, sometimes one minute at a time.

Focus on the Possibilities

Learn to focus your energy on the positive and ask yourself: What can I learn from this experience? Where are opportunities for personal growth? You probably envisioned one particular story of how your life would unfold, but there are other paths too. When you come upon a roadblock, consider it an opportunity for new possibilities.

Awaken New Dreams

Listen to your heart. Late at night or in the quiet morning hours, what is your heart telling you? What dreams lie dormant? Follow your heart and you will realize other desires or visions to pursue.

Meditate

Meditation has incredible health benefits, including reducing stress and fatigue. There are many forms of meditation as it is practiced by many different religions and spiritual traditions. The goal of meditation is to calm your thoughts, cultivating a relaxed and peaceful state of mind. Set time aside to meditate each day, as it will help you heal your mind, body, and spirit.

Be Thankful

Did you know that being thankful is the number one factor affecting your happiness? Even when your dreams are not realized, be thankful for the blessings you experience each day. Write them down in a journal and review them often. Did you wake up breathing? Be thankful. Do you have a roof over your head? Be thankful. Do friends and family surround you? Be thankful.

Embrace the Process

I am still mourning and reflecting on what happened, and contemplating what it will be like without children or grandchildren as I get older. Sometimes I even wonder who will inherit my fine china and jewelry collection. My aunt Maxine advised me to enjoy my china and jewelry everyday. She encouraged me to unpack and to use my great-grandmother's embroidered napkins. I've decided to quit worrying about what happens when I die. There's really no point in saving anything or tucking it away in a cedar chest. That's one thing that three failed pregnancies have taught me—to live in the present moment and count my blessings rather than my losses.

Popular culture tells us that we can have it our own way. That's a joke. The challenge is to accept disappointment and allow it to shape your character in positive ways. When you get to that point where you can let go—let go of what you want, let go of demanding to have your way—that's the moment you know you've found inner strength and peace.

Even though my dreams of starting a family have not been realized, I still believe that my life has meaning apart from being a mother. Throughout my life I've had a lot of desires. As a child, I wanted to be a writer and live in a cottage on the beach with my desk facing the ocean. That desire has somewhat materialized. I live one mile from the beach and my desk faces west. I can also take my laptop to the beach to write. We may not receive all of our heart's desires, but we can be thankful for what we have. Learn to focus on the positive. Pain is inevitable, but misery is optional.

CHAPTER SEVEN
family and friends

Infertility brings crisis into the immediate and extended family. It not only affects the infertile couple, but also their grandparents, parents, and siblings. When a crisis occurs in the family each person is affected on various levels, because the family is an emotional unit. The difference between each person is his or her ability to manage oneself and one's contribution to the family.

When family members don't share the common experience of infertility, they may react with unsolicited advice. "You should lose 20 pounds, and then you'll get pregnant." "You wouldn't have miscarried, if you hadn't smoked when you were a teenager." "You just need to relax and take a vacation." "Maybe you aren't meant to be a parent." "If you haven't had a baby by now, don't you think it's time you gave up?"

Their advice is hurtful and their comments may strain the family relationships. Without familial support, the infertile couple feels isolated when experiencing a miscarriage, tubal pregnancy, or a failed medical treatment. Their loss, although deep and profound, is invisible to their family members. Infertility often highlights a family's inability to deal with problems. Further, when a new family crisis arises such as an ill grandparent, the infertile couple's struggle may be overshadowed. Without a frame of reference, family members may use coping techniques that alienate the infertile couple. They may cutoff, blame, or deny what's happening. Again, each family member's response to crisis depends upon his or her ability to manage oneself.

Family members also have the potential to be great encouragers to one another. Infertility may bring the family closer together as they bond to create a support system for the infertile couple.

When Lisa experienced a stillbirth, she and Michael relied on their family for emotional support. Their family even arranged a memorial service for their baby. Because their family acknowledged their loss and showed compassion, Michael and Lisa felt understood and validated in their difficult time of despair.

Knowing Who You Are

My family and friends think of me as a daughter, sister, granddaughter, niece, cousin, and friend. I am all those things, but I am also a mother. My babies, or fetuses to be technically correct, didn't live very long, but I still think of them often. When their intended birth dates roll around every year, I remember them and wonder what they would have looked like. My hazel eyes or Brian's blue eyes? Blonde or brunette? Fair or olive complexion? I will never forget them.

To My Fellow Friends with Infertility

We all share the same pain, regardless of our varied experiences. Some of us achieved pregnancy naturally or through ART, and for different reasons the pregnancies didn't work out. Some of you, regardless of your efforts, have not been able to conceive. There are also women and men who struggle with infertility before or after having their own biological child. The details of our stories may differ, but we share common ground. We know the challenges of trying to achieve a pregnancy and the heartbreak of not being able to sustain it.

Through this book, I hope to encourage you, because I know how easily fears and depression can turn into feelings of hopelessness. Infertility is overwhelming and it's easy to lose yourself in the midst of countless medical appointments, ultrasounds, and blood draws. Stay centered. Take time out, when needed, to care for yourself.

Dealing with Other People

I'm a fairly private person, so I don't advertise my fertility troubles, especially when I'm around people I don't know very well. For example, I play tennis with various groups of women who are more acquaintances than friends. Naturally, between games, we chat about life and work. In the normal flow of conversation the same question pops up, "Do you have kids?" I always shy away from the inquiry because some women ask for details. Others overreact. Some look at me, horrified, and say things like, "I'm so sorry. You must feel depressed. That's just awful."

I know they're trying to show compassion and relate to me. I appreciate their efforts, but it can be uncomfortable when everyone's eyes are on me. I play tennis to escape my fertility problems. It's my outlet. I forget everything when I'm on the courts. My mind is focused on sending an ace over the net, putting backspin on the ball, and nailing a lob with perfect execution. While on the courts, I certainly don't want to discuss my pregnancy losses and infertility issues.

Some women pry, asking all kinds of personal questions because they're curious. I understand why. Most of them have children and don't know what it's like to experience a tubal pregnancy. Women with children are in the majority. Only 1 in 20 women in the United States have infertility issues. I'm one of the special 1 in 20, so naturally other women want to know my story. Women bond through sharing their experiences and listening to one another. It's how we form relationships, but I'd rather talk about where we grew up or which university we attended. That would be an easier and lighter conversation.

Michelle's and Suzanne's Stories: Dismissive People

Most people don't understand infertility. They don't realize it's a medical condition. It's like having diabetes or arthritis. It can't always be cured and, more than likely, you'll have to live with it. Because of people's ignorance, they can be insensitive. I've met strangers who were dismissive about my pregnancy loss. One time

I met a nurse while having my blood drawn. She asked why I was doing the blood test. I explained that I'd had a tubal pregnancy and the blood test was to make sure my hormone levels were dropping after a recent laparoscopic surgery. She had no obvious response to my story. It appeared as if she wasn't really listening. I think she was just filling the silence with her words as she pushed a large needle into my vein.

It's understandable that strangers would have little interest in someone's pregnancy loss, but Michelle was upset when her friends simply ignored her feelings.

> *None of my friends could relate to me. They avoided me and quit calling. They never said a word to me or my husband about our loss. They were dismissive about my miscarriage. They never knew my baby, so I guess it didn't seem real to them.*
>
> *To make matters worse, none of the ladies or ministers at my church called me to see how I was doing. Not one single person. I was angry with our church in general because they failed to do anything. They are Christians and are supposed to help each other and bear one another's burdens. They never reached out to us. It was hurtful.*
>
> *Then, three weeks after we lost our son, I got a baby shower invitation from a friend. I was so angry and upset, because we were grieving. She knew I had just lost a baby and never even contacted me, except to send the baby shower invite. It was totally insensitive.*
>
> ### ~ **Michelle**

Normally, friends and family have the best intentions. They always want to help and offer a kind word, but sometimes they struggle knowing what to say. I try to give them the benefit of the doubt when the words they say hurt my feelings. After my third pregnancy loss, my good friend said, "Lesley, maybe you weren't meant to be a mother." I'm sure she never intended to upset me and was only trying to help, but her words felt like a dagger piercing my heart. She knew I had been trying to have a baby for years. She has children of her own. I wondered, *How could she say that to me?* Throughout my struggle, I had shared my journey with her. Hearing her words shocked me into silence. I wanted to ask her, *What kind of a jerk do you think I am?* but gave her the benefit of the doubt.

Well-meaning people of faith have said things such as, "God never gives you more than you can bear." They are obviously not walking in my shoes. This statement sends me over the edge. I know for a fact that God gives us a whole lot more than we can bear. A one-liner like that provides no comfort. No guidance. No wisdom. No help. Maybe they mean well, but it's tough to stomach that kind of statement when you feel as though you're walking through hell without a bucket of water.

> *Women are made to feel like they're overreacting if they grieve the loss of an unborn child. It's a very silent grief for so many women who feel that they can't grieve publicly.*
>
> *So many people pushed me to get over it. Three months after my miscarriage I was still struggling. People just kept telling me, "You just need to move on."*
>
> ~ **Suzanne**

Patricia's and Amy's Stories: Words That Don't Help

Besides the insensitive, uninformed comments I've already mentioned, here are other things you hope you'll never hear:

- "You just need to relax."

- "It'll happen."

- "Let nature take its course."

- "It's a good thing you miscarried. You might have had a Down Syndrome baby."

- "At least you miscarried at sixteen weeks. It's a good thing it didn't happen in the third trimester."

When I miscarried at sixteen weeks, my family and friends didn't think of it as a "real" baby yet. They thought it was good that my miscarriage happened early as opposed to later in my pregnancy. They didn't understand why I was so upset. I had to explain to them how quickly a fetus grows from week to week. I showed them pictures to prove my baby already had arms and legs. My baby was perfectly formed already. He had fingers and toes. He had little eyebrows, eyelashes, and hair on his head. His teeth and bones were growing, and he could even suck his thumb. I had heard his heartbeat at several ultrasounds. Other people don't know what it feels like to lose a baby that early in a pregnancy. I was very sad for a very long time.

*~ **Patricia***

- "Something good will come out of this."

- "If you haven't had a baby by now, maybe it's time you just gave up."

- "It was God's will."

- "It's been a long time since you lost your baby. Don't you think it's time to move on?"

- "My friend got pregnant on vacation; maybe you should take a trip."

- "Everything is going to be fine."

- "You just need to lie down and hold your legs up in the air after you have sex."
- "You already have one child, isn't that enough?"

> *I miscarried at eighteen weeks. Afterwards, I got up out of bed because of the two kids I already had. I knew they needed me. Just because I have children doesn't mean I don't grieve the baby I lost. People act like I don't have the right to be sad about my miscarriage. They don't know what it feels like. They have no right to judge me.*
>
> *~ Amy*

To Family and Friends Wanting to Help

It's tough knowing the right thing to say to someone who is struggling with a pregnancy loss or infertility. Of course you want to be supportive and give your loved one encouragement in the midst of his or her crisis. You have the best intentions but might not know how to help. Often your presence is the best medicine and shows your care.

Some men and women may feel guilty after a pregnancy loss or once they are diagnosed with infertility. It's easy to get caught up in "what-if" scenarios, so try not to say things that sound as if you are placing blame. For example, avoid saying things like, "Well, if you weren't a smoker." or "I hear being overweight contributes to fertility problems. Maybe you should lose 20 pounds." or "You should exercise more."

Encouraging Things You Might Consider Saying

Without a similar experience, you won't have an easy time making sense of someone else's suffering. If you can't think of something positive to say, don't say anything. Silence is okay. Don't offer advice when you have no idea what the other person is experiencing. Here are some positive and affirming things you might want to say to your family member or friend:

- "I am sorry for your loss."

- "Is there anything I can do for you?"

- "I don't know what to say, but my heart goes out to you."

- "This must be a difficult time for you."

- "I am here for you."

Bonnie's Story: Practical Ways to Help

If you want to be a trusted and thoughtful friend or family member, consider the following guidelines for helpful things to say and do:

- Respect your friend's privacy. Don't discuss your loved one's situation with outsiders unless you receive permission.

- Be thoughtful. Call before showing up unannounced at your loved one's home or work.

- Prepare a casserole or baked goods to deliver to your friend. If you're not a cook, order take-out from your favorite restaurant. Comfort food is always good.

> *An older woman in my neighborhood called me, out of the blue, two months after I lost Stephen, my baby that I miscarried at thirteen weeks. She said, "I've just made chili and I thought you might enjoy some of it."*
>
> *That was the sweetest thing anybody ever did for me. I started crying because I was having an emotional day. It meant so much that she thought of me and brought me dinner.*
>
> ~ **Bonnie**

- Offer to do chores. Imagine a pile of laundry staring you in the face when all you want to do is crawl under the covers and sleep for days. Take the initiative and help your loved ones by cleaning their house and doing the laundry. Just loading the dishwasher is helpful.

- When you grocery shop, call your friend to ask what she might need from the store.

- Suggest a low-key outing to help get her mind off the loss or fertility problem.

- Just listen. Don't pass judgment or give advice.

- Allow your friend time to heal. Don't try to rush her through the grieving process.

- Know your own limitations. If your friend seems depressed and your efforts are not helping, or if you don't know how to help, encourage your friend to seek out a professional counselor. Sometimes a helpful suggestion can steer a person back on the road to recovery.

CHAPTER EIGHT

what now?

Six years. Three failed pregnancies. Shattered dreams. Unending grief. Drained emotions. Strained finances. And it's still not over. Brian and I continue to talk and work through our thoughts and feelings regarding the detour from how we expected our lives to unfold as "mommy and daddy," lives perfectly planned for a son and a daughter. Normal expectations. Because our reproductive hopes have vanished, we must transition to the healing stage and answer for ourselves, "What now?"

Vacillating. Adrift on waves of mixed emotions. Understanding just out of reach, making the private experiences of infertility so very hard to communicate. It feels like our world is ripping apart and we are left with no lifeline—just questions. Why can't we have babies like everyone else? What's wrong with us? What will we do now? Will we do IVF again? Will we have regrets 10 years down the road if we don't try IVF one more time? Will we hire a surrogate? Will we adopt? Will we live childfree? How will we ever be happy again?

With so many questions swirling overhead, we feel overwhelmed. We fear making the wrong decision. Knowing the statistics, the risk of having a baby with birth defects scares us. Should we gamble once again with Mother Nature? Is a 20 to 30 percent chance worth spending another $15,000 for IVF, when failure is such a great possibility?

Every decision we make about ART has consequences. Just like with other choices in life—choosing a career and a spouse—we lose something and we gain something.

Because of our mixed emotions regarding our reproductive choices, we will have internal conflicts whatever we decide. That's why every answer creates a new struggle.

In an effort to sort it out, Brian and I put our list-making skills to work. We explored the pros and cons of having children. Thinking through our choices helped us connect with our motivations and made our decisions more tangible.

Our options to proceed or cease and desist in our family-making endeavors include:

Pros of Having Children

- Our contribution to the world. Growing our family. Raising responsible children to help make this world a better place to live (sounds goofy, but it's true).

- Long-term security. Our children would help take care of us (hopefully) when we get old.

- Inheritance. Having a child would give us an heir to receive whatever money we might have when we die and the child would be the recipient of our possessions and family heirlooms, including three sets of fine china, a jewelry collection, hundreds of cassette tapes from the '80s, CDs from the '90s, three shoeboxes filled with vintage baseball cards, and handmade surfboards.

- Our lives would be enriched by having more people in our life to love.

Cons of Having Children

- We would have less time to pursue personal interests and career goals.

- There is physical pain associated with delivery.

- Kids would drain our bank account.

- We would travel less.

- Being a parent means being in a constant state of worry about the children's well-being.

- At our age, the risk of having a child with birth defects is increased.

According to the March of Dimes, women over the age of 35 have an increased risk of delivering a baby with a birth defect. Down Syndrome and autism are two common defects that increase as the mother's and father's ages increase. Even with young moms there are no guarantees. The risk for Down Syndrome:

Age 25, 1 in 1,250

Age 30, 1 in 1,000

Age 35, 1 in 400

Age 40, 1 in 100

Age 45, 1 in 30

Age 49, a 1 in 10

Options for Future Baby-Making Endeavors

- Avoid fertile days altogether and say, "Forget it!"

- Alleviate stress and don't time anything; just have sex whenever we want and don't worry about trying to get pregnant. Of course, I am at a higher risk of having another ectopic since I've already experienced two.

- Just do "it" around ovulation time, hoping for a miracle.

- Use an ovulation kit to time our baby-making activities.

- Try IVF again, at a cost of about $15,000.

149

My first experience with IVF was all consuming. It was a strict regime. I took prescription medications, endured daily injections, had weekly blood draws, stayed on bed-rest, and underwent countless ultrasounds. It wasn't a normal or fun way to live.

Despite the rigorous routine, the thought of doing IVF one more time is tempting. It is my only option to have a biological child. When I miscarried during my first IVF cycle, I had a strong urge to sign up for one more treatment. Like so many women, I was pumped up on hormones and thought anything was possible if I just tried hard enough. Fertility treatments can be likened to a carrot that dangles just out of reach. It's easy to believe that, if you run fast enough, you'll snatch the carrot and make it across the finish line with a baby in your arms.

I remember telling Brian, "We could do IVF again in three months, as soon as my body has recovered from the miscarriage." In the midst of my disappointment, I was determined and wanted to force a pregnancy to work. I sought to be in control of the situation. I had the innate desire to create new life even at the expense of my own health. My maternal longing was driving me, as was an overwhelming sense of failure. I wanted to "succeed" at being normal!

"Let's not jump into another IVF cycle right away," Brian replied.

We took a step back for a year, discussing our options and debating pros and cons. For us, the emotional trauma of three lost babies had taken a toll. We were exhausted at the prospect of attempting another IVF cycle and unenthusiastic about trying to get pregnant on our own, knowing a tubal pregnancy could occur.

As time passed, we gradually decided not to do IVF again. The pros turned into maybes and no longer outweighed the cons: expensive, slim chance for success, high risk for birth defects, likelihood for depression, and inevitable weight gain.

The Last Straw

Fast forward three months. Brian and I attended a Fertility

EXPO as research to write this book. At the event, we won a complimentary consultation to meet with one of the best fertility specialists in Southern California. Because the appointment was free, we decided to go to find out what our chances would be if we did IVF again.

As soon as Brian and I sat down in Dr. X's office she asked, "How can I help you?"

Not wanting to hog the conversation, I kept silent and looked over at Brian, giving him the chance to talk.

"We've done IVF once and it was unsuccessful. At this point we're both 40 and want to know what our chances are if we tried again," he explained.

"Did you get pregnant with IVF before?"

I jumped in with details. "Yes, I got pregnant with IVF but miscarried at ten weeks. I now know that I have a hormone imbalance, but we don't know why I had the miscarriage."

"Well, we'll need to run more tests," she said reviewing my medical records. "If we transferred three blastocysts, you'd probably have a 30 percent chance of getting pregnant. I would take an aggressive approach with your IVF cycle. You also need to be monitored more often since you have hormone imbalances. We will need to do blood tests and a new semen analysis to know for sure. Lesley, you should have an ovarian reserve test so we know how many eggs you have left."

We talked to Dr. X for an hour about our history. She explained that her focus was not only to get me pregnant but to care for me while pregnant.

Dr. X asked, "Lesley, do you want to do IVF again?"

"I'm not sure. There's a lot to consider and the odds aren't in my favor," I said.

"Brian, how do you feel?"

"Well, I really want to have kids, but I'm not sure if it's worth the emotional and mental strain of going through IVF again. If it didn't work out, that would be really tough for us to take. Of course, our chances are even lower this time because we're both 40, so that makes a big difference."

"I'm also concerned about the high risk of having a baby with birth defects. At our age we have a 1 in 100 chance," I added. "Honestly, I don't think I want to commit to doing another IVF cycle."

"Well, think about it. If you decide to do IVF again, I suggest you do it in the next couple of months, before you turn 41," Dr. X added.

The Morning After

The next morning Brian and I sat quietly, hands wrapped around our ritual morning cups of coffee. I was barely awake as he asked, "Well, what do you think about the appointment with Dr. X? How do you feel about doing IVF again?"

"I didn't think it was a topic that needed to be addressed. I thought we had already made our decision back before the Fertility EXPO."

"Well, now that we've seen a new doctor, I was wondering if you'd changed your mind."

I felt the muscles in my neck tense up and a feeling of dread came over me. "Have you changed your mind? Are you telling me you want me to go through the emotional roller coaster of IVF again, when we only have a 30 percent chance?"

"No, I'm not saying..."

By this point I was nervous. Fear and a renewed sense of failure filled every vein in my body as I practically screamed at Brian, "If you don't want to do IVF, why would you ask me what I thought? You should damn well know by now what I think about the topic. Do you really want me to go through that physical hell again? Do you want me to lose my mind and fall back into depression and even deeper grief? Do you want our sex life to suffer again and let some doctor tell us when we can and can't do it? Do you want to throw $15,000 down the drain again?"

"Sorry, honey. I didn't mean it that way," Brian said, as he tried to back off.

"Well, yesterday when you told the doctor that you 'really wanted kids' I wondered if you suddenly wanted me to do IVF again. If we don't ever have children, are you going to be okay with that? Do you want to divorce me and find some 20-year-old to have your babies?"

"No, honey, we're in this together. There's no one person to blame. You have tubal problems. I have sperm problems. I want kids, but we made our decision not to try any more treatments. Given what we've been through, I really don't want us to go down that path."

"Well, last time you wanted to gamble and play the odds with a 40 percent chance that IVF would work. Why don't you want to do IVF this time with a 30 percent chance? You like to gamble, why don't you want to roll the dice again?"

"I want my wife to stay healthy and sane. I'm not asking you to go through it again. You did it once and that was enough. I don't want to go through the emotional turmoil either. It's not worth it. We've been through enough."

Ovarian Reserve Test

It was only normal that our emotions would vacillate about our decision to quit using ART. Some days we felt confident of our decision and other days we wavered. In an attempt to assure ourselves that we had made the right decision, I submitted to one last blood test to check my ovarian reserves. Although not 100 percent accurate, the blood test is an indicator of the quantity of eggs in the ovaries.

I hoped the test would give us an idea of how likely I was to get pregnant on our own. Even though I wasn't planning to do IVF, I still wanted to know about the health of my ovaries. Secretly, I also thought that the test would somehow vindicate me by showing that my ovaries are actually healthy.

The doctor called with my ovarian reserve test (ORT) results saying, "Lesley, your blood tests show that you have a poor ovarian reserve. I'd like to see your numbers over 10. A 7 is considered low, and you tested at 3.2, so I would use an aggressive treatment plan for you, if you decided to go forward with IVF."

I knew "an aggressive treatment plan" would mean hyperstimulating my ovaries to force them to produce more follicles. If it worked, everything would depend on the number of eggs I produced and how many were fertilized with Brian's sperm. So many unknowns. The blood test was discouraging. I saw no point in putting myself through IVF again, when the chances were so slim.

Seeking Psychological Help

I grew tired of trying to figure things out on my own. The circular thinking was exhausting. "Maybe I should." "No, I shouldn't." "Well maybe." "No!" Eventually, I sought professional help. Jumping right into the middle of my torment, I asked the psychologist, "How do I get to a place where I am at peace about not doing IVF again, and be done with the whole fertility thing and just live my life? How do I silence my mind, quiet my dreams, and give up my desire to have children?"

"It's a process," she said, pushing her little black glasses up on her nose.

"Process is good, but I need to gain some traction," I replied.

The doctor encouraged me to consider various options and outcomes. "Try it on," she suggested. "What would it feel like if you did one more cycle of IVF? Would it give you closure, knowing you tried one last time? Or would going through the emotional, financial, and physical challenges overwhelm you too much? Imagine the various scenarios and see how it would feel to you. How would you feel if IVF worked and you had a baby? How would you feel if IVF didn't work and you didn't get pregnant or lost the baby during the pregnancy? Try it on."

I spent weeks trying on "what-if" scenarios. Pure emotional gymnastics, but it helped me sort through my feelings and thoughts. I pushed forward seeking closure, needing peace. I realized that I was pressuring myself and needed to let go of my own and other people's expectations. Counseling helped me take ownership of my decisions. Finally, I gave myself permission to ignore other people's advice and opinions. I awakened to the fact that my opinion was the only one that mattered.

Standing firm in my convictions, I began trusting my instincts, listening to my heart and inner spirit. When life becomes hectic, it can be difficult to hear the small voice of wisdom from within, but I made the effort to stop and listen. I have always believed that the heart is the wellspring of life. And my heart was quietly telling me to let go and quit trying to control the situation.

Hearing my counselor say, "You are normal," was the best medicine. Those three words validated my experience and told me I wasn't crazy for being "indecisive." Experiencing pregnancy loss and infertility was not just about the loss of my ability to have children. It was multiple losses. Loss of three pregnancies. Loss of feeling normal. Loss of control. Loss of a future with my baby. Loss of a first holiday. Loss of celebrating birthdays. Loss of carrying on our family legacy. Loss of being like my friends and family who have kids.

Experiencing that much loss left me feeling abnormal, inadequate, and less than a fully functioning woman. Quitting my job after my third pregnancy loss gave me some form of control in my life. Part of my acceptance was to take charge and drastically change my career path.

My losses have changed me, but they don't make me a loser. Through the journey, I have learned that I am more than my inability to have children. Today, I can say I am normal. What I feel is normal. I am not ashamed. My infertility is a part of my physical condition, but it does not define me. It does not limit me. I am more than my fertility.

Considering Your Options after ART

When ART is no longer an option, there are other family-building choices you may wish to consider, such as donor eggs/sperm, surrogacy, adoption, and living without children (aka childfree). Each individual and every couple has different goals and limits. Technology is a wonderful thing, but with it comes the burden of making difficult decisions without knowing a definitive outcome. Even with the best doctors, it's a gamble, and you must be willing to take the risks. Each decision is very personal and varies from person to person. There are no right or wrong answers.

Elizabeth and Paul's Story: Donor Eggs

For five years Elizabeth and Paul struggled trying to have a baby. She got pregnant twice the old-fashioned way, but both pregnancies ended as ectopics. Then, Elizabeth and Paul tried five cycles of IVF, spending over $75,000 without success. Determined to have a baby, Elizabeth decided to take matters into her own hands and find an egg donor.

> *"Paul, I want to pursue finding an egg donor. Then, I want to do another round of IVF to try again for a baby."*
>
> *"You're just making a spontaneous decision. Elizabeth, you haven't thought this through. "*
>
> *"That's not true. I don't feel like I'll be missing out on anything by using an egg donor. I'm the one who will be carrying and delivering the baby, and it will be with your sperm. So, I have thought it through."*
>
> *"Well, what if I don't agree to it?"*
>
> *"If you don't agree, then we need to start divorce proceedings immediately, so everything can be settled before September. I'm planning to do my transfer in September. I'll use donated sperm if I have to. If you're not in this with me, I'll move back to New York to be around my family and friends. I know where I'll work, and I've been looking at houses in New York. I'm serious. I've really spent a lot of time on this."*
>
> *"I think it'll be hard on you being a single mother. Have you thought about that?"*

"Yes, that's why I'll move back to New York, to be around my family. They'll help me."

"If this IVF cycle doesn't work, how do I know that you're not just gonna kick me to the curb and push on with your plans without me?"

"I promise you that this will be our last IVF cycle. After this, I will not bother you about it ever again. We will remain married and go about our happy little lives."

"You're putting me through hell over all this."

"Well, you're the one who said that, when I put my mind to something, I do it. So, this should come as no surprise to you."

"Elizabeth, I want to stay married to you. I'll agree to using an egg donor, but I don't want to know anything about who the donor is going to be. Don't tell me her name. Don't tell me where she's from or anything about her. I don't want to see pictures of her. Just make sure she looks like you, at least as close to you as possible. That's all I ask."

"Okay, I'll take care of it."

~ Elizabeth and Paul

Elizabeth knew in her heart that she was meant to be a mother. During her acupuncture treatments she could visualize her babies. She felt her babies around her. Determined not to give up, she searched for the perfect egg donor, looking at hundreds of Los Angeles and San Diego agencies.

After checking out Southern California agencies, I even talked to a woman in New Jersey who specializes in Jewish donors. Most of her girls are from Israel. I come from a strong, traditional Jewish family. We celebrate Jewish holidays like Yom Kippur. It's always been a big part of my life. So, in the beginning of my search, I wanted a Jewish donor. I thought it was really important. I quickly found out that Jewish donors are hard to find and much more expensive than non-Jewish donors.

I took a lot of time interviewing the donor agencies because they are all very different. Some offer videos of the girls, and some focus on their test scores, talents, and schooling. There are also private agencies that spend a lot of time with each girl to understand why she wants to be an egg donor, making sure she's emotionally ready.

I finally decided to stay close to home to save money. If I chose an Israeli girl, I would have to fly her out for the egg retrieval, adding to the overall expense.

Through the egg donor-recipient evaluation process, I realized that I didn't need a Jewish donor. I'm Jewish and the baby would be mine. I was going to give birth to this baby, therefore, the baby would be Jewish and growing up in a Jewish home. My husband is not Jewish, but he's very supportive.

When looking for a donor, I didn't want someone who had features, talents, or characteristics that stood out because I would be able to see those characteristics in my baby. I considered a girl who was an opera singer. But I knew that if my baby was born with a beautiful voice, I would associate that with the opera singer.

I kept going back to this one donor who seemed like an average girl. She was pretty, had good parents, wanted to be a nurse, had decent SAT scores, and was in college. She and I had a lot of the same hobbies, and we had the same birthday. She was half Hispanic and half German, and she had green eyes with blonde hair. I'm German and have blonde hair and blue eyes. I got the chance to see pictures of her siblings and her parents, and learned about her grandparents' history. It seemed like, physically, she would be a really good match, and we shared similar characteristics. Paul's side of the family is Hispanic and his father has very blue eyes. There are a lot of blue eyes on his side of the family. So I thought that there would be a chance of us having blue-eyed babies with fair skin. Maybe some blonde hair, so they would look like me. If not, then the babies would look like Paul, and that would be fine. For me, picking a donor was about calculating what the baby might look like, which was really important.

~ Elizabeth

Although Paul didn't want to take part in finding an egg donor, he was interested in understanding how the egg donor process worked.

"Elizabeth, like I said, I really don't want to see photos of the egg donor, but I would like to know how this is going to work. At what point do I come into the picture?"

"Well, once I find the right egg donor, the doctor will give her hormone-boosting shots for about a month. The hormones will stimulate her ovaries to produce a high number of eggs. I hope this will give us twelve to fifteen eggs."

"That sounds like a lot."

"Not really. Sometimes the eggs aren't actually viable. So, I just hope we'll get enough so we can have five or six healthy embryos. We'll freeze whatever embryos we don't use. I'll take hormone shots to synchronize my cycle with the egg donor's cycle. When it's time for the donor to ovulate, they

use IVF procedures to retrieve the eggs from the donor's ovaries. Then, you'll give a sperm sample, with which the doctor will fertilize the donor eggs. At that point, it will be just like the last IVF cycle we experienced. On day five the doctor will transfer two of our embryos into my uterus. Hopefully, one of the embryos will implant in my uterus and I'll be pregnant."

~ Elizabeth and Paul

Elizabeth and Paul were happy when the doctor retrieved fourteen good eggs from their egg donor, all of which fertilized into embryos. The doctor transferred two of the embryos into Elizabeth's uterus and froze the other twelve.

I stayed home relaxing and doing nothing during the post-embryo transfer phase, hoping for the best. The two embryos that we transferred took. I couldn't believe it. I was so excited.

My doctor confirmed that I was definitely pregnant. My hCG level was 525, so I suspected immediately that I had twins.

To make a long story short, I went into premature labor at thirty-five weeks. Since I was having twins, my doctor performed a C-section. I was thrilled when my baby girls were born with fully developed lungs. It was truly a miracle that Paul and I had two healthy, beautiful girls.

~ Elizabeth

Elizabeth and Paul needed time to adjust to the fact that they used another woman's eggs with his sperm to create their babies. In the beginning it was a little awkward for both of them. On a few occasions Paul referred to the egg donor as the "biological mother."

It really devastated me when Paul called our egg donor the biological mother of our children. One day I finally told him, "You can't refer to her as the biological mother. She truly is just a donor and that's all she is. I am the one who carried my babies for nine months and I'm the one who birthed them."

After having my twins, I had weekly sessions with a therapist for a long time. She helped me feel more comfortable about having used an egg donor. I remember her saying, "Elizabeth, I have to believe that your body fluids are in your baby girls. For months they were swimming within your womb. There's got to be something from you that gets into your babies." Her words helped.

The twins look just like Paul. They both have blue eyes. Katie is very fair and has blond hair. Dawn has a little bit darker hair with olive skin. They really don't look anything like the donor. That helps. I got lucky.

One thing that still bothers me is that my mother tells me all the time, "The babies don't look anything like you."

I try my best to ignore her comments. I never told my mother that I used donor eggs and I never plan on telling her.

I love Katie and Dawn as if they were my own flesh and blood. I am still glad we used donor eggs because, without them and the wonders of technology, I wouldn't have my beautiful girls.

Paul now understands that family is what you make it. He stopped mentioning the donor and it makes me feel much better. We're a real family now and we're very happy.

~ **Elizabeth**

Sarah and Matt's Story: Surrogacy

We all have different experiences, leading us to make different choices. Sarah took birth control pills for fourteen consecutive years, beginning at 18 years old. At 32, she and her husband Matt decided it was time to start a family, so she quit taking the pill. She expected her body to adapt and produce a normal menstrual cycle.

After being off the pill for fourteen months, Sarah still hadn't gotten her period. Her OB-GYN explained to her that the birth control pills had stopped her ovaries from ovulating. Sarah knew that, even if her cycles were regular, her chances of getting pregnant would drop by 50 percent by the time she turned 35. Armed with this knowledge, she and Matt decided to take an aggressive approach to building their family. They chose to use a surrogate.

Matt and I didn't want to go through life without children. We felt like we would be missing out on something if we didn't have a family. We had already tried IUI and IVF, but those procedures didn't work for us, so we chose surrogacy. Even if I couldn't carry a baby, I really didn't want to miss out on motherhood. It was more important for us to focus on the bigger picture of having a family rather than how we got a family.

Luckily, we were able to use my eggs and fertilize them with Matt's sperm. During fertilization we didn't get as many embryos as we had hoped—only four. Two embryos stopped growing. One embryo was fragmented. Only one perfect embryo remained. So, the doctor transferred the perfect embryo and the fractured embryo into our surrogate's uterus. Then we waited.

When our surrogate was on bed rest after the embryo transfer, I took care of her three children during the day, while her husband was at work. I cooked meals, cleaned her house, and washed their clothes. It was the least I could do.

As it turned out only one embryo implanted in our surrogate's uterus, but we were happy it worked. Luckily, our surrogate had an easy pregnancy. When she started having contractions, she quickly went from 5 cm to 6 cm and, with each contraction, she dilated one more centimeter until she got to 9 cm. Matt and I were in the delivery room with her every step of the way. When the doctor told her to push, she gave two pushes and our baby girl was out. The delivery was truly amazing!

~ Sarah

Although it's often assumed, using a surrogate does not guarantee having a full-term pregnancy and live birth. The success rate for surrogacy depends on several factors: the age of the woman contributing the eggs, the quality of the sperm, the age of the surrogate and her ability to conceive, the experience of the doctor, and the fertility clinic's IUI and IVF success rates.

Most people use a gestational surrogate, also called the "host method" or "third party reproduction." Doctors use a modified IVF cycle to suppress the surrogate's body from ovulating. Then, at just the right time, the doctor transfers the embryo(s) into the surrogate's uterus. Success rates depend mostly on the health of the egg(s).[13]

Rachel and Steve's Story: Adoption

Choosing adoption starts with both individuals being honest about their personal views. Steve told Rachel that he viewed adoption as raising someone else's child. He also feared that the biological parents of an adopted child might change their minds. He didn't want someone yanking his adopted baby out of his arms. Rachel desperately wanted to be a mom, no matter what challenges they had to overcome. She was willing to take any risk.

After Rachel's miscarriage and four failed ART cycles, Steve finally agreed to try adoption as a means to build their family.

We chose an open adoption because we wanted to give our child access to information about his birth family. Adoption is quite expensive and a long process. We didn't know how long it would take the agency to find a baby for us, once the application was completed.

A few weeks after the paperwork was filed, I had a brain aneurysm and subsequent brain surgery. Then, two weeks after my surgery my father passed away. It was a very traumatic time. I kept wondering how I would take care of a newborn, because I was taking anti-seizure medicine and grieving over the death of my father. I called the adoption agency to talk to them about my situation.

The timing of everything worked out. A few months later, the agency called to tell us about a baby boy who was up for adoption. It was a rape and the girl was in her teens. The girl had been adopted by her aunt because her mother lived on the streets. After we agreed to adopt her baby boy, Steve and I met the girl. She asked me to be in the birthing room so the baby would imprint on my voice and touch.

I had never seen a birth before, and I don't do well with blood. It was hard to watch. I felt uncomfortable, like I was in someone's bedroom. The last thing I wanted to do was see the birth mom's "you know what."

When she birthed him, the umbilical cord was wrapped around his neck, so he was blue. Patting him hard, the nurses put him immediately into the incubator. I wanted the birth mom to hand me the baby, but she didn't want to touch him.

When my husband handed me the baby for the first time, I felt guarded because I knew the birth mom could still change her mind. Her aunt, uncle, sister, and a few friends were gathered around, watching the delivery. We also knew that her grandmother and brother didn't want her to give up the baby for adoption.

Later that night Steve and I went back to our hotel. We were in shock yet elated at the same time. It was hard to believe—and difficult to let ourselves feel—that this adorable, sweet baby could be the final realization of all our hopes and dreams.

After all the paperwork was complete, we were allowed to take our new baby boy home. We were a little petrified because we had no experience. We wanted to be good parents but didn't know what to expect.

When Joseph was two months old, my sister passed away. I remembered thinking, "God did not save me from the aneurysm and a life of disappointment for nothing. He's got great things planned, Joseph being one of them."

God's timing of giving us a baby was so perfect. It was so hard to deal with my father's passing and all the stuff that needed to be done with his estate and belongings. My sister passed on the same day that my father's estate closed. I then had to go back to the probate lawyer and open another probate for my sister.

I thought I was going to crumble under the pressure and stress but, looking at my baby, I realized that I couldn't sit around in the past wallowing in grief. I needed to feed Joseph in two hours. The grief needed to be dealt with, very much so, but I had to take care of my baby's needs.

I wanted a baby so bad, but if we didn't get one then Steve and I planned to travel. My view of life is that if you get lemons, just make lemonade. I don't focus on the dark side of things. I'm inclined to focus on the blessings.

My baby didn't come in the way I thought it would happen. Looking back, I made a very bad decision to have an abortion as an 18-year-old girl. When I look down and see the scar, I am reminded of a bad decision I made so many years ago. But now, I know that God can completely turn around a bad situation and bless me beyond my imagination, with my child, who says, "Mommy, I love you." When he's hurt he says, "Mommy, hold me."

In the future, when Joseph asks about his birth mom, we will tell him that his birth mom was not equipped to be a mom and she took great care in picking his future family. We will tell him that he didn't come to us through my womb but through our hearts.

Adopting a child comes at great costs. It's complicated because so many people are involved. You don't get to celebrate it fully, in a way. I imagine it would be like someone who has a history of miscarriages and then finds out she's pregnant. She doesn't really feel like she can celebrate it until the baby is there. Your joy gets robbed. You don't get to say, "I'm pregnant. Isn't this fabulous and wonderful."

The way our life has unfolded is not how we would have chosen it in the beginning, but now we have so much joy and fulfillment. Our family has been completed in a better way than we could have ever imagined."

~ Rachel

Kelly and Tom's Story: Living Childfree

Kelly and Tom have always loved children. They volunteer in a tutoring program, helping kids with homework, and play key roles in the lives of their eight nieces and nephews. After Kelly and Tom completed their PhDs they decided to have children of their own.

For a long time Kelly's periods were irregular and accompanied by abdominal pain. An ultrasound showed six fibroids growing in and around her uterus. One fibroid was the size of a grapefruit and another was the size of a tennis ball. Her doctor suggested a hysterectomy, but Kelly refused and insisted on keeping her uterus, hoping she could still have children.

During surgery to remove the fibroids, the doctor realized the fibroids had grown stems attached to Kelly's uterus, making removal even more difficult. She was advised not to get pregnant following surgery, because it was unlikely that she would be able to carry a baby to full term and could even bleed to death with complications.

> *After surgery, I was very disappointed and wondered if I should have tried to get pregnant sooner instead of finishing my PhD. For a long time I was very upset, but I have learned that we can't get everything we want in this life. Tom and I talked about other options, such as adopting a child. We thought about it for a long time, but we never felt a desire to adopt.*
>
> *Our friends and peers asked, "Why are you not going to adopt?" They thought that with so many children in the world who need good home, we would make great parents. We told them that we didn't feel adoption was the right choice for us.*
>
> *I think a lot of people assume that something is wrong with you if you don't have children. Then, they pass judgment and act like something is wrong if you are not adopting, especially when you have the*

resources to do it. I think many people give in to that peer pressure, but Tom and I feel strongly that we are not supposed to adopt.

We are following our hearts in our decision, even if that means living without children. We believe that when one door closes a window will open up with other opportunities. Tom and I have very fulfilling lives. We get a lot of satisfaction out of volunteering with children and spending time with our nieces and nephews. We are very content and happy.

~ **Kelly**

Life without Children

Most women tell me that they cannot imagine their lives without children, and that's what motivates them to continue fertility treatments. That's why they get a second and even a third mortgage on their homes to pay for medical expenses.

I can imagine my life without children. I have lived without them for decades. Granted, I will miss the idea of having a family with Brian. The financial burden, emotional stress, and physical gymnastics of ART drove me to the limits of what I'm willing to endure. I am done. I will live childfree. It's not my ideal situation, but I have accepted my reproductive limitations and will live with the gifts I was given.

The God Question

For a long time I struggled asking, "Why isn't God answering my prayers to have children?" I wondered how God was involved. I questioned God's role in my ability to procreate. Finally, I came to the conclusion that God is not to blame for my reproductive limitations. In other words, I don't think God made me infertile. I am equipped with reproductive organs just as I am endowed with a pancreas, liver, and stomach. Infertility is a medical condition. For example, I wear glasses because I can't see road signs at a distance when driving. God didn't cause me to be nearsighted any more than he caused my infertility. My eyes are weak. My reproductive organs are weak. Both problems are medical conditions. Nothing more, nothing less.

Angry with God

A number of men and women have confided in me that they are angry with God for taking their babies. I have been angry at times too. It's okay to be angry with God when you don't know what to do with your raging sorrow over the deep loss you've experienced. It's normal to be angry. You won't go to hell for getting angry.

Pregnancy loss and infertility are an overwhelming burden to bear. Go ahead and blame God, because Almighty can take it. I don't believe God will hold it against you. I've said my fair share of negative things to God, even screaming at the Creator a time or two and I'm still standing. I believe God understands the depth of our pain and has compassion for us when we grieve.

My Choices

For me, being pregnant is one of the best parts about having children. I loved being pregnant, having my little baby growing inside my belly. If I am going to have children, I want to be able to carry the pregnancy to full term and give birth. I want the entire experience, not just the end result. I want the risks and joys to be all mine. I don't want to be in the position of blaming another person if my baby died while on their watch, and I would. For these reasons, I choose not to use a surrogate. It can be a beautiful experience for some, but I don't feel comfortable making that choice.

Almost every person I know who has adopted children is passionate about their decision. Adoption is a great option for many couples. Since having biological children is important to Brian and me, we have chosen not to adopt or to use donor eggs or embryos.

There are moments when my resolutions crumble and I question our decision to stop trying to have children. Since I can't hold my babies, sometimes I melt when I see a cute little baby playing on the beach. I imagine how fun it could be to build sandcastles with my own children. I would love to hear their giggles and see their smiling faces.

I was a mother for only a short time, but I am thankful to have had the experience of being pregnant. I refuse to live a bitter and resentful life because of my losses. Each day I focus on the positive things in my life, such as the love of family and friends. I choose to live in my blessings, create good out of my sorrow, and be an "encourager" to others.

> *I always felt like Lesley and I would be great parents and imagined taking my son to ball games, teaching him how to throw a ball, and helping with his homework. But after years of trying and failing, and especially after the pain of the last pregnancy loss, I have resigned myself to the fact that we won't ever have kids. Although it works out great for many people, adoption and surrogacy are not appealing to me. More rounds of IVF seem like slim odds for a child and high odds for more pain and disappointment.*
>
> *A life without children gives us more time, money, and emotional energy for other things. Now, it's up to Lesley and me to look forward, dream a little bigger, and take a few more risks. Life won't necessarily be better or worse than we had imagined, only different.*
>
> **~ Brian**

Personal Reflection

I still believe in the power of prayer, even though God hasn't answered my prayers to have children. I still believe God performs miracles, even though I don't have a little miracle to hold. I still believe God heals, even though my left fallopian tube doesn't function properly.

Because there are so many factors beyond my control, I have

relied on prayer. Sadly for me, my prayers have not been answered in the way I desired. But even though I didn't get what I wanted, my life is still meaningful. I have my health, food, shelter, love, and the ability to dream new dreams.

My goal is to be spiritually open and mentally flexible when I encounter another sharp curve in the road. I will carefully navigate the twists and turns until my path is straight and clear again. When I face another switchback, I will focus my energy on the positive and ask: "What can I learn from this experience? Where's the opportunity for personal growth?"

Along my journey, I have experienced grace, peace, and hope to carry me through the tough days. I am fortunate to have phenomenal people around me to encourage me, make me laugh, and give me a shoulder when I needed to cry. For all these blessings, I am grateful.

Kelly's Story: A New Purpose

Good moms and dads make parenting their purpose and calling. They put all their energy into raising their children as best they can, giving them every possible advantage in life. Most parents would sacrifice their lives for their kids.

Everyone wants to have a worthwhile reason for living. The question many infertile men and women ask themselves is: If I don't have children, then what's my purpose in life? This is a hard question, especially if you don't have a job or career that motivates and inspires you. If being a member of the Mommy Sorority or Daddy Fraternity isn't an option, then what's your purpose in life?

> I've asked myself, "What is the purpose of my life?" Now that I can't have children, my purpose is different—not a less-than or greater-than—just different. I have accepted that I have a purpose in my life, other than having children, and it's a very fulfilling life. I have gained a sense of peace with that realization.

> *If you can't let go and say, "I have to have..." or "I won't be happy if I don't have children," then I think you're putting obstacles in the way of experiencing peace and contentment. Allowing the absence of having a baby and trying to control the situation then can be stumbling blocks to personal and spiritual growth. I don't have it all together all the time, but I try to grow from each experience and find the good in each situation. You can be happy if you choose to be.*

~ Kelly

Create Meaning Out of the Crisis

Remember, you are more than your fertility. Your life is not just about procreating. You are endowed with a wonderful intellect, giving you the ability to choose and chart new courses in your life. You don't have to be confined by failed expectations. You can envision a new dream and bring it to fruition.

The key to overcoming obstacles is to create meaning out of the crisis. You have the wherewithal to rise above any difficulty. Your reproductive system does not have to define you. You are more than your fertility.

There are hundreds of worthwhile causes, and some of them may even ignite a new fire under your feet. Maybe you feel as if you've lost your purpose in life because your family isn't exactly the way you pictured it would be. Don't lose heart. Have no fear. Regardless of where you are on your journey, rest assured that you will find a renewed purpose in life. In time, you can reconnect your passion with a new vision for your life and work.

You Are Normal

You may question whether or not you are normal, but you are. Whatever you feel is normal for you. There's no shame in having strong emotions over reproductive disappointments. It's normal to feel sadness, numbness, fear, anger, guilt, loneliness, disgust, anticipation, or a host of other emotions.

Though our journeys differ, we are on the same path. My way is not the only way nor is it the "right" way for you. Whatever you think and feel is normal for you. Whatever decision you make is yours alone to make. You get to do it your way and on your own timeline. You have permission to choose the path that best suits you: not your mother, not your neighbor, not your best friend.

Read, question, and seek counseling for guidance, not to get it right, but to do it your way. You don't have to please anyone but yourself. You don't have to rise to a particular standard other than the measure you've determined for yourself. You have the power to choose your path, whatever that may be. When you pick your path and name it, you will feel empowered and in control of your life once again. It takes time to arrive at such important decisions, but the knowing will give you peace and confidence.

There's power in saying: "I choose to do IVF." "I choose not to use ART." "I want to adopt." "I choose not to adopt." "I want to use a surrogate." "Surrogacy is not for me." "I am ready to live childfree." Whatever you choose to do is right for you. Pick your path and make no apologies. If you make a choice, it is the right one for you.

In the Meantime

While you navigate the twists and turns throughout your journey, take time each day to be aware of the blessings you enjoy. Be present in the moment. Be amazed by a beautiful sunset. Smile when you see a rainbow overhead. Take note of the things you appreciate and love. Write them down in a journal and review them often.

Focus on everything that is right, good, pure, and lovely. Following any traumatic experience in your life, being grateful is the number one factor affecting your happiness.

Never Giving Up

I believe my heart's deepest desires will be fulfilled because I won't give up on life.

There are always other options. I will find new dreams to pursue and other talents to perfect. I am grateful to be living in a time and place where I can do whatever I desire—continue my education, serve as a volunteer, launch a new career, start a new business, or live a simple life.

In the midst of fertility challenges and obstacles that are beyond my control, I choose to focus on the positive, things that are honorable, true, and inspiring. I believe there's more to life than what I can see, hear, smell, taste, and touch on this earth. This divine knowledge gives me hope that there's a bigger plan unfolding before me.

My Prayer

Spirit come
Indwell this heart of mine
For I am imperfect
Limited without your light
Divine, lover of my soul
Breathe in me
And I will soar to new heights
With purpose and conviction
Strength and knowledge
Deeper wisdom
Learned through hardship and tears
My thorns have taught me
Patience, peace, understanding and love
I am transformed
Now renewed
I lift my eyes to heaven
And give thanks once again
Holy, holy, holy is the Lord God almighty
Who was, who is and who is to come.
Amen.

BIBLIOGRAPHY

(1) Chandra, Anjani, Martinez, Gladys M., Mosher, William D., Abma, Joyce C., & Jones, Jo. (2005). "Fertility, Family Planning, and Reproductive Health of U.S. Women: Data from the 2002 National Survey of Family Growth." Centers for Disease Control and Prevention. Hyattsville, Maryland.

(2) Sepilian, Vicken P. "Ectopic Pregnancy." eMedicine Online. 7 May 2010. <http://emedicine.medscape.com/article/258768-overview>.

(3) "What Causes an Ectopic Pregnancy?" American Pregnancy Association Online. September 2009. <http://www.americanpregnancy.org>.

(4) Reddy, U. M. (2007). "Recurrent Pregnancy Loss: Nongenetic Causes." Contemporary Ob/Gyn, 63-71. Michels, T. C. & Tiu, A. Y. (2007). "Second Trimester Pregnancy Loss." *American Family Physician*, 76(9), 1341-1346.

(5) Youran, D. B., Bopp, B. L., Colver, R. M., Reuter, L. M., & Adaniya, G. K. (2008). "Acupuncture Performed before and after Embryo Transfer Improves Pregnancy Rates." *Fertility and Sterility*, 90, 240-241.

(6) Chang, Raymond, Chung, Pak H., and Rosenwaks, Zev. "Role of Acupuncture in the Treatment of Female Infertility." American Board of Oriental Reproductive Medicine Online: 2009. <http://www.aborm.org/research/research.16.infertility.pdf>.

(7) Orloff, Judith. "The Health Benefits of Tears." *Psychology Today*. 27 July 2010. <http://www.psychologytoday.com/blog/emotional-freedom/201007/the-health-benefits-tears>.

(8) "Vasectomy Reversal Success Rate Factors: Will a Reversal Work?" Vasectomy Online. 2009. <http://www.vasectomy.com/ArticleDetail.asp?siteid=R&ArticleId=5>.

(9) "Male Infertility: Causes." Health Communities Online. 1998-

2010. <http://www.urologychannel.com/maleinfertility/causes.
shtml>.

(10) "Male and Female Infertility." <u>Mayo Clinic Online</u>.
2010. <http://www.mayoclinic.com/health/female-infertility/
DS01053>.

(11) "Census Bureau Projects U.S. Population of 308.4 Million
on New Year's Day." <u>U.S. Census Bureau Online</u>. 2009. <http://
www.census.gov/newsroom/releases/archives/population/cb09-
201.html>

(12) "Age and Fertility: A Guide for Patients." <u>American Society
for Reproductive Medicine Online</u>. 2003. <http://www.asrm.org/
uploadedFiles/ASRM_Content/Resources/Patient_Resources/
Fact_Sheets_and_Info_Booklets/agefertility.pdf>

(13) "Report on Gestational Surrogates and Live Birth Rates."
<u>Society for Assisted Reproductive Technology Online</u>. 1999.
<http://www.sart.org>.

GLOSSARY

Acupuncture - the procedure of inserting and manipulating needles into various points on the body to relieve pain or for therapeutic purposes.

Acupuncturist - a healthcare professional who is qualified or professionally engaged in the practice of acupuncture.

Antibiotic - medicine that kills infections caused by bacteria.

Assisted Reproductive Technology (ART) - any kind of fertility treatment where both the egg and sperm are handled in a lab.

Azithromycin - antibacterial medicine that is prescribed to treat bacterial infections in many different parts of the body.

Bacteria - tiny organisms that live in and around your body. Some bacteria are good for your body, and others can make you sick.

Birth Control - also called contraception or family planning. Things you can do to keep from getting pregnant. Using a condom and taking a birth control pill are examples of birth control.

Birth Defects - problems with a baby's body that are present at birth.

Blastocyst - A blastocyst is a highly differentiated, highly developed embryo that has grown to the point where it is ready to attach to the uterine wall (implantation). In naturally conceived pregnancies, the egg is released from the ovarian follicle and picked up by the fallopian tube where it is fertilized by sperm. The resulting embryo starts out as a single cell, which then must grow and differentiate until it has the capacity to attach to the uterine wall and connect to the mother's blood stream. The embryo divides from one cell into two cells, then four cells, eight cells, 16 cells, etc. until it reaches several hundred cells at the time of implantation and reaches the blastocyst stage on day five or six after ovulation.

Blastocyst transfer - transfer of an embryo to the uterus after it has been allowed to grow in the laboratory for five days to the blastocyst stage, as opposed to three days, which is typical for a standard IVF procedure. A blastocyst transfer is a technique incorporated with in vitro fertilization (IVF) designed to increase pregnancy rates and decrease the risk of multiple pregnancy.

Bleeding (also called spotting) - when blood comes out of the vagina during pregnancy.

Bravelle - is the brand name of a follicle-stimulating hormone (FSH). The hormone is used to stimulate the ovaries to make multiple follicles which normally contain one egg each.

Braxton-Hicks contractions - contractions that help prepare your body for labor. They are different from labor contractions because they don't get stronger or happen faster over time. They also may stop when you move around.

Clomid or Clomiphene (kloe' mi feen) - is a commonly used fertility drug to induce ovulation (egg production) in women who do not produce ova (eggs) but wish to become pregnant. Clomid is in a class of medications called ovulatory stimulants. It works similarly to estrogen.

Down Syndrome - a congenital disorder that occurs when an individual has three, rather than two, copies of the 21st chromosome. This additional genetic material alters the course of development and causes the characteristics associated with Down syndrome. The incidence of births of children with Down syndrome increases with the age of the mother. But due to higher fertility rates in younger women, 80% of children with Down syndrome are born to women under 35 years of age. Down syndrome is the most commonly occurring chromosomal condition. One in every 691 babies is born with Down syndrome. (Source: National Down Syndrome Society)

Doxycycline - an antibiotic that is effective against many infections.

Ectopic Pregnancy - occurs when the fertilized egg attaches itself in a place other than inside the uterus. Almost all ectopic pregnancies occur in a fallopian tube, and are thus sometimes called tubal pregnancies. The fallopian tubes are not designed to hold a growing embryo; the fertilized egg in a tubal pregnancy cannot develop normally and must be treated. Up to 1 pregnancy in 50 is ectopic, which means "out of place."

Embryo - a fertilized egg that results when an egg and sperm combine. The embryo implants itself into the wall of the uterus and grows to become a fetus.

Estrogen - a female hormone that causes eggs to develop in the ovaries and be released.

Fertility Specialist - also called a reproductive endocrinologist. A medical doctor who is an expert in helping women get pregnant.

Follicle stimulating hormone (FSH) - A follicle-stimulating hormone test measures the amount of FSH in a blood sample. FSH is produced by the pituitary gland. In women, FSH helps control the menstrual cycle and the production of eggs by the ovaries. The amount of FSH varies throughout a woman's menstrual cycle and is highest just before she releases an egg (ovulates). In men, FSH helps control the production of sperm. The amount of FSH in men normally remains constant. The amounts of FSH and other hormones (luteinizing hormone, estrogen, and progesterone) are measured in both a man and a woman to determine why the couple cannot become pregnant. The FSH level can help determine whether male or female sex organs (testicles or ovaries) are functioning properly. (Source: WebMD.com)

Genetic disorder - any disorder caused, wholly or in part, by a fault or faults in the inherited genetic material within a person's cells that is, in the genes formed from the DNA which make up the chromosomes in a persons cells.

Genetic screening or testing - techniques used to test for genetic disorders, involve direct examination of the DNA molecule itself. Genetic tests are used for several reasons such as: carrier screening, which involves identifying unaffected individuals who carry one copy of a gene for a disease that requires two copies for the disease to be expressed; preimplantation genetic diagnosis; and prenatal diagnostic testing.

Guided imagery - a program of directed thoughts and suggestions that guide your imagination toward a relaxed, focused state. You can use an instructor, tapes, or scripts to help you through this process.

Hashimoto's Thyroiditis - an autoimmune disease in which the thyroid gland is gradually destroyed by a variety of cell and antibody mediated immune processes. It was first described by the Japanese specialist Dr. Hashimoto Hakaru in Germany in 1912.

Hysterosalpingogram (HSG) - an X-ray test that looks at the inside of the uterus and fallopian tubes and the area around them.

Infertility - defined as not being able to get pregnant despite having frequent, unprotected sex for at least a year. Ten to 15 percent of couples in the United States are infertile.

Immunizations - process by which an individual's immune system becomes fortified against an agent.

Intra cytoplasmic sperm injection (ICSI) - used when the sperm have a difficult time penetrating the eggs. Using a needle the embryologist places one sperm in each egg.

Intrauterine Insemination (IUI) - a procedure in which sperm are "washed" to separate them from the semen and inserted via a small tube into the uterus around the time of ovulation after the ovaries have released one or more eggs. The hope is that the sperm will swim into the fallopian tube and fertilize an egg resulting in pregnancy.

In Vitro Fertilization (IVF) - is the process of fertilization by manually combining an egg and sperm in a laboratory dish. When the IVF procedure is successful, the process is combined with a procedure known as embryo transfer, which is used to physically place the embryo in the uterus.

Lupron - a hormone administered before the period is expected to start. Used to prevent premature ovulation.

Maya Abdominal Massage - an external non-surgical massage that affects the digestive and reproductive organs.

Methotrexate - may be used in the treatment of ectopic pregnancies, which allows the body to absorb the pregnancy tissue and may save the fallopian tube, depending on how far the pregnancy has developed.

Miscarriage - is the term used for a pregnancy that ends on it's own, within the first 20 weeks of gestation. Most miscarriages occur during the first 13 weeks of pregnancy. Miscarriage is the most common type of pregnancy loss, according to the American College of Obstetricians and Gynecologists. Studies reveal that anywhere from 10-25 percent of all clinically recognized pregnancies will end in miscarriage. Chemical pregnancies may account for 50-75 percent of all miscarriages. This occurs when a pregnancy is lost shortly after implantation, resulting in bleeding that occurs around the time of her expected period. The woman may not realize that she conceived when she experiences a chemical pregnancy. (Source: American Pregnancy Association)

Multiple gestation pregnancy - a twin or triplet pregnancy. Approximately 2 percent of all pregnancies produce twins.

Ovarian hyper-stimulation syndrome - a condition in which you ovaries may become swollen and painful as a result of taking hormonal medications that stimulate the development of eggs.

Ovidrel - a hormone that induces ovulation when the follicles are mature. It is injected 36 hours before an egg retrieval.

Ovulation - The release of an ovum (also known as an oocyte, female gamete, or casually, an egg) from the ovary.

Oxytocin - a hormone secreted by the posterior pituitary gland. Oxytocin is released during labor, helping to facilitate birth and ejection of milk.

Patency - the openness (lack of obstruction) of a bodily passage or duct.

Prednisone - an oral, synthetic (man-made) corticosteroid used for suppressing the immune system and inflammation.

Progesterone - a steroid hormone produced in the ovary; prepares and maintains the uterus for pregnancy.

Qi - means "life force" or "energy." According to Chinese philosophy, Qi is thought to be inherent in all things.

Selective reduction - the practice of reducing the number of fetuses in a multifetal pregnancy (those involving more than one fetus).

Stillbirth - is defined as the intrauterine death and subsequent delivery of a developing infant that occurs beyond 20 completed weeks of gestation. Stillbirth occurs in about 1 in 200 pregnancies. The majority of stillbirths happen before labor, whereas a small percentage occurs during labor and delivery.

Testicular Sperm Extraction or Retrieval - a sperm retrieval procedure that is either performed through the skin (percutaneous) or through a small opening in the skin about half-inch in size. Sperm can be gathered from the epididymis, a sperm rich tube at the back of the testis. Testicular Sperm Extraction involves removing small samples of testis tissue for processing and eventual extraction of sperm.

Transvaginal egg retrieval - a procedure designed to remove eggs from the ovaries.

Viability - capable of normal growth and development.

ABOUT THE AUTHOR

Lesley Vance has a B.A. in Communications and an M.A. in Ecumenical Theology. For over 15 years, she has worked as a Public Relations Consultant for a wide range of clients in the areas of publishing, education, entertainment, health care, and high tech. She leads an infertility support group as a volunteer for RESOLVE, the National Infertility Association, and is a contributing writer for *San Diego Family Magazine*. Lesley writes a blog about infertility on her website, www. lesleyvance.com, and resides in Encinitas, California with her husband. Infertility Journeys is her second book.

To contact the author, write to:

Lesley Vance
c/o Duck Hill Press
P.O. Box 236142
Encinitas, CA 92023

Email Lesley and read her blog on her website at:

www.LesleyVance.com

NOTES

www.ingramcontent.com/pod-product-compliance
Lightning Source LLC
Chambersburg PA
CBHW071223290326
41931CB00037B/1858